UNDERSTANDING DRUG TREATMENT IN MENTAL HEALTH CARE

The Wiley Series in

CLINICAL PSYCHOLOGY

J. Mark G. Williams
(Series Editor)

School of Psychology, University of Wales, Bangor, UK

Further titles in preparation: *a list of earlier*
titles in the series follows the index

UNDERSTANDING DRUG TREATMENT IN MENTAL HEALTH CARE

Alyson J. Bond
and
Malcolm H. Lader
Institute of Psychiatry, University of London

Foreword by Dr David Wheatley

JOHN WILEY & SONS
Chichester • New York • Brisbane • Toronto • Singapore

Other Wiley Editorial Offices

John Wiley & Sons, Inc., 605 Third Avenue,
New York, NY 10158-0012, USA

Jacaranda Wiley Ltd, 33 Park Road, Milton,
Queensland 4064, Australia

John Wiley & Sons (Canada) Ltd, 22 Worcester Road,
Rexdale, Ontario M9W 1L1, Canada

John Wiley & Sons (Asia) Pte Ltd, 2 Clementi Loop #02-01,
Jin Xing Distripark, Singapore 0512

Library of Congress Cataloging-in-Publication Data

Bond, Alyson J.
   Understanding drug treatment in mental health care / Alyson J.
Bond and Malcolm Lader.
       p.   cm. — (The Wiley series in clinical psychology)
   Includes bibliographical references and index.
       ISBN 0-471-94227-8 (cloth : alk. paper). — ISBN 0-471-96171-X
   (alk. paper)
       1. Mental illness—Chemotherapy. 2. Psychopharmacology.
   I. Lader, Malcolm Harold. II. Title.   III. Series.
       [DNLM: 1. Mental Disorders—drug therapy.   2. Psychotropic Drugs—
   pharmacology.   WM 402 B711u 1996]
   RC483.B66   1996
   616.89'18–dc 20
   DNLM/DLC
   for Library of Congress   96-1090
                                                                        CIP

British Library Cataloguing in Publication Data

A catalogue record for this book is available from the British Library

ISBN 0-471-94227-8 (cased)
ISBN 0-471-96171-X (paper)

Typeset in 10/12 Palatino by MHL Typesetting Ltd, Coventry
Printed and bound in Great Britain by Biddles Ltd, Guildford and King's Lynn
This book is printed on acid-free paper responsibly manufactured from sustainable forestation,
for which at least two trees are planted for each one used for paper production.

CONTENTS

ABOUT THE AUTHORS

Alyson Bond is a Senior Lecturer and Chartered Clinical Psychologist at the Institute of Psychiatry. She has researched into the effects of drugs on emotions and psychological processes and the treatment of anxiety disorders and she is particularly interested in the combination of drugs and psychological therapies. Her current research interests include the relationship between the biological and psychological aspects of hostility and aggression. She has published numerous articles in international journals on these topics.

Malcolm Lader is Professor of Clinical Psychopharmacology at the Institute of Psychiatry, University of London. He is also an Honorary Consultant Physician at the Bethlem Royal and Maudsley Hospitals. He holds a research appointment on the External Scientific Staff of the Medical Research Council (unlimited appointment). He has researched for over 30 years on various aspects of psychotropic medication. Although the bulk of this work is concentrated on the benzodiazepines, he has also contributed numerous publications on antidepressants, hypnotics and antipsychotic medication. He has over 550 publications plus 12 written books and 15 edited books. He is a member of the editorial boards of over twenty journals.

FOREWORD

For many decades I have been involved in the evaluation of psychotropic drugs, firstly in primary care and latterly in hospital. The advances in techniques have been great indeed, but frustratingly not matched by correspondingly significant therapeutic improvements. Rather the present state of advancement is one of quality than quantity: we still have to wait for two to three weeks before our depressed patients even start to respond to drug treatment and even then response may be but partial and incomplete. On the credit side, drugs are safer and better tolerated so that patient compliance is improved. We must also rely on as much help as possible from psychological techniques to offer our patients the best possible chances for alleviation of their ailments. The purpose of this book is to survey the state of the *whole* art, the integration of psychotherapeutic interventions with drug treatment.

In the 1960s, we had effective drugs to combat most of the major psychiatric disorders: anxiety, insomnia, depression, mania, schizophrenia and epilepsy: we did not have a treatment for Alzheimer's disease — and we do not now. Clinical trial methodology at that time must appear crude compared to the sophisticated techniques of today. Measures of improvement were often confined to a simple estimate of how much better, or worse, the patient might feel. And yet the former is the clinical aim of treatment and its proof, as Alyson Bond and Malcolm Lader point out, has been evidenced by the rapid acceptance of psychopharmacology as the cardinal treatment for psychiatric illness. It is with a feeling of some unease that I view the present state of clinical trial methodology. Thus the increasing demands for voluminous documentation, admittedly necessary for drug registration purposes, may prove a distraction to the detriment of accurate clinical observation. Now that proven treatments are available for most psychiatric disorders, the scientific need for placebo controls may conflict with the strictures of that hallowed addendum to all trial protocols: the Declaration of Helsinki. At a time when Ethics committees are paying more and more attention to this aspect of research, we may have to rely increasingly on drug–drug comparisons.

One of the most important areas for psychotropic drug use is primary care. Indeed, the general practitioner can diagnose and treat most of the affective disorders. But does he have the time or the training so to do? Very often this is not the case and this book may well help to fill this gap. But the average practitioner in this sphere of medicine is unlikely to be familiar with the refinements of the various psychotherapeutic approaches that are available to the clinical psychologist as an adjunct to psychopharmacology. Once more this volume succinctly reviews the issues involved. The hospital-based psychiatrist, on the other hand, is in a much stronger position to provide total care for his or her patients. Nevertheless, psychotherapists will surely welcome the essentials of psychopharmacology that are outlined in this book and psychopharmacologists may the better understand the supplementary benefits that psychotherapy has to offer. There is an increasing realisation of the importance of psychological influences in physical disorders involving important specialities such as: cardiology, immunology, dermatology, allergology and gynaecology to mention but a few. No one specialist can embrace the whole of medicine and needs a volume such as this to augment knowledge when dealing with the mental component of physical disorders.

Depression is a prime example of a psychiatric disorder that may be involved in many medical disciplines. As the authors of this book go to some pains to emphasise, explanation to the patient is of prime importance to successful case management and nowhere is this more important than when treating this illness. For indeed depression is an illness and this must be impressed on patient, spouse, family and friends alike. A personal experience illustrates this, the patient being a lady from the provinces who had suffered from chronic depression for most of her life. She responded extremely well to a six-month course of an antidepressant and radiantly commented: 'for the first time in 20 years my husband realises that I have been ill'. No greater compliment could one wish for.

Many psychiatric disorders have psychosocial components and here the primary care physicians are at an advantage, benefiting from an intimate knowledge of their patients' circumstances. The many stresses of life do indeed constitute 'the slings and arrows of outrageous fortune', which I studied for many years when I was in charge of the Maudsley Stress Clinic. I was particularly interested in the impact of the many stresses that constitute an inescapable component of everyday life, on the mental and physical well-being of my patients. Hardly surprising perhaps that I found some 50% of patients developed depression in response to long-continuing stressful circumstances. By treating the depression, it was often possible to break the *vicious circle* whereby stress initiated depression, which in turn perpetuated the inability to cope with it.

The true value of this book lies in its eclectic approach to the treatment of psychiatric disorders through the integration of the humanistic and scientific aspects of patient care. It will provide an invaluable aid to all those who combine their efforts to help the mentally ill.

David Wheatley MD, FRCPsych
Royal Masonic Hospital, London

SERIES PREFACE

The Wiley Series in Clinical Psychology aims to provide a comprehensive set of texts covering the application of psychological science to the problems of mental health and disability. The series includes books written by clinical psychologists for their own colleagues and for other health professionals. But it also includes books written by other mental health professionals where the topic is of interest to all who seek to take an applied science approach to mental health and illness.

The most commonly used approach to mental health problems is psychotropic medication. Whether we are a medical student or junior doctor learning about psychiatry for the first time, a GP or GP trainee, a psychologist doing cognitive therapy, a social worker visiting a distressed family, or a psychiatric nurse running a group on a psychiatric unit or doing a home visit, many of the people we see will be on psychotropic medication. All health professionals need to know about such medication, whether or not they are responsible for prescribing it. The problem has been to know where to start, and this book is written to meet this need. What psychotropic medication is available, and what is commonly prescribed? How do they have their effects? What determines whether a medical practitioner prescribes, and what determines adherence by patients? How can adherence be improved?

The authors take the reader systematically through each of these questions, and provide a book that will be as useful a summary for the expert as it is an introduction for the novice. They take account of the fact that mental illness and distress is multifactorially determined, and do not exclude psychological and social factors in considering aetiology, maintenance and treatment. Against this context, their comprehensive review of pharmacological approaches will prove of great benefit to all of us who have responsibility for the welfare of people with mental health problems.

J. Mark G. Williams
Series Editor

PREFACE

Drug treatment forms an important part of the care for those with mental health problems. Generally, as the severity of the disorder increases, the greater the likelihood that drug treatment will prove necessary. This does not preclude their use as temporary relief or as an adjunct to other social or psychological treatments in those with less pervasive disorders. As the number of drugs with differing and complex actions increases, the more difficult it is for mental health professionals, especially those who are not prescribers, to keep abreast of these developments. General practitioners are increasingly being expected to prescribe for patients with mental health problems, yet they are not psychiatrically trained. It is important that all those involved in patient care have some knowledge of the actions of these drugs, the indications for their use and the manner in which they are prescribed. The intention of this book then is to describe how, why and when drugs are used alongside other treatments in mental health care. In the first two chapters we describe the history and general principles of drug treatment and how drugs are classified. Then in Chapter 3, we discuss some social and psychological aspects, such as why doctors prescribe and patients' attitudes to psychiatric care. In Chapter 4 we describe the way in which drugs act on the human body and the effects of the body on the drug. Drug development and the importance of evaluating new treatments are also discussed. Drugs affect not only mood but cognition and behaviour and they are often used with other treatments. In Chapters 5 and 6 we discuss ways in which drug effects can be examined and the evaluation of comparative and combined treatments.

In the rest of the book we have adopted a problem orientated approach. Thus one chapter is devoted to each main group of mental health problems, e.g. anxiety, depression, schizophrenia, and the drug treatment of each is described along with other non-drug treatments which have been validated. A further chapter is devoted to other problems which the professional is likely to encounter. Space did not allow us to be more comprehensive and so some areas like dementia have had to be omitted.

Chapter 1

INTRODUCTION

People have always used psychotropic substances to alter mood. However, the study and therapeutic use of mind-altering drugs is a relatively recent phenomenon. The major developments in psychopharmacology (the study of drugs used to treat mental health) took place 40 years ago. The prototypes of all the major groups of psychotropic drugs were discovered then. They followed in the wake of other physical treatments in psychiatry, such as deep insulin therapy, psychosurgery and electroconvulsive therapy. Since the introduction of effective drug treatments, the management of patients with psychiatric disorders has changed radically. Fewer patients now need long-term hospital care, treatment has shifted to out-patient or community care and there has been a tremendous growth in our understanding of the factors leading to psychological malfunctioning and the actions of psychotropic drugs.

Conversely, people have become worried by the increase in biological treatments for psychological disorders. Historically the other physical treatments were regarded as a cure-all and were grossly over-used. Eventually this led to the abandonment of one (deep insulin therapy) and severe restrictions on the other two. Thus, drug treatment has also come to be regarded with suspicion. People now justly express concern about issues such as side-effects and dependence. However, this may lead to the prescription of subtherapeutic and therefore ineffective doses, the under use of new compounds or stopping treatment too soon.

Drugs are an essential part of mental health care. It is therefore extremely important that all health-care workers are informed about the uses, advantages and drawbacks of psychotropic drugs and their possible interactions with other treatments. Psychotropic drugs do not cure psychiatric disorders. They suppress distressing symptoms and behaviour until natural remission takes place. If a drug is prescribed in too low a dose, it will be deemed ineffective, in too high a dose, then side-effects will be intolerable and if it is stopped prematurely, then symptoms may reappear. Many psychotropic drugs do not act immediately. It may take two to four weeks for their therapeutic action to be seen and progress may not be even, some symptoms improving long before others. Explanation and reassurance about such factors are important to aid the patient's understanding and adherence to any treatment regimen.

Prescribing always takes place in a social context. It is not just the patient who is affected by a psychiatric disorder. Family, friends and colleagues also have to cope with his/her disturbed mood and behaviour. Treatment has consequences for them too and their needs and attitudes need to be considered. The support of those close to the patient is very important to the success of any treatment and without such support progress can easily be undermined.

A drug can never be prescribed in isolation. It is always the result of an interaction between doctor and patient and therefore psychological factors are pertinent. A good doctor-patient relationship increases the likelihood of drug treatment being successful. The simplest form of psychological treatment is non-judgemental support but explanation of possible causes and symptoms and reassurance about recovery aid the patient's understanding of his/her condition. Treatment should be regarded as collaborative, the doctor and patient agreeing on the goals.

It is important to recognise that drugs are not the only treatment for psychiatric disorders. Psychological treatments are used alongside or instead of drug therapy. The foundations of psychiatry and psychology are rooted in totally different methodologies which has led to problems in the past. However, the two approaches can be, and often are, used together in clinical practice. Understanding the best way of integrating the two is paramount to the successful treatment of patients suffering from psychological distress.

Chapter 2

GENERAL PRINCIPLES OF DRUG TREATMENT

In this chapter, the current models of psychiatric disorder are described. Despite their differing origins and emphasis all have the common belief that psychiatric disorders do exist and patients with them need treatment. Because drug treatment is based on diagnosis of a psychiatric disorder, the principles and method of psychiatric diagnosis are discussed and then a brief history of the development of psychopharmacology and a current classification system are outlined. Many different factors contribute to a psychiatric disorder resulting in a variety of conceptual models and treatment approaches (Figure 2.1).

Historically psychiatric disorder has been viewed in various ways. One prevalent belief was that the individual was possessed of an evil spirit, a devil or the ghost of an ancestor. There have been swings between this spiritualistic and the medical concept through the ages, resulting in either punishment or treatment but sometimes with little difference between them for the

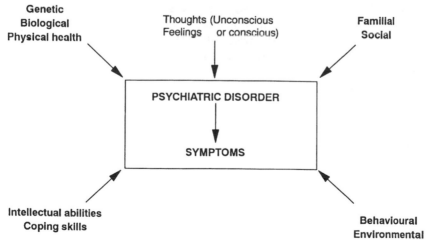

Figure 2.1   Factors contributing to a psychiatric disorder

individual concerned. There are many biblical accounts of the possession of devils but the times of the ancient Greeks were generally tolerant of psychiatric problems. The more scientific medical approach was then founded in attempts to understand the brain and mental processes. However, the Middle Ages showed a reversion back to the belief in evil spirits and horrific punishments. Eventually the Christian church saw itself as offering mercy and a refuge for those suffering from these conditions but it was not until the 14th century that the 'insane' started to be commonly segregated from Society into institutions. These early ideas started to develop into the forerunners of different models in the 19th and early 20th centuries.

MODELS OF PSYCHIATRIC DISORDER

Various models are currently used in psychiatry because of the history of the discipline and the different backgrounds of the practitioners. It is therefore important not only to recognise these but to try and integrate them logically within a multidisciplinary approach. There are currently six main models of psychiatric disorder (Table 2.1).

The Disease or Biological Model

As psychiatry developed from medicine, it is not surprising that the disease model predominates and that depression and schizophrenia, for example, are frequently described as mental illnesses. The use of drugs as treatment tends to reinforce this relationship as drugs are used to cure or improve physical illnesses. According to the disease model which recently has also become known as the 'biological' model, psychiatric disorder occurs as a consequence of physical and chemical abnormalities or changes in the body, primarily the brain, and drugs or other physical treatments like ECT may be used to normalise these changes. The notion of an illness implies that there is a fundamental difference from normal, and a categorical rather than a dimensional approach is therefore

Table 2.1   Current models of psychiatric disorder

Biological or disease
Psychodynamic
Behavioural
Cognitive
Social or interpersonal
Humanistic

preferred. For the illness to be diagnosed, a clinical syndrome must be identified. This is done by observing and interviewing the patient. A physical examination may also be done but the aim of this is to exclude the presence of any physical illness rather than to confirm the presence of a mental illness. The examination of clinical state has, however, the same aim of scientific objectivity as the diagnosis of a physical illness and a certain diagnosis implies a certain type of treatment. The patient is regarded as a passive recipient of treatment to cure the illness or at least to control the condition and thus remove the distressing symptoms. The psychiatrist has an authoritarian role as a consultant in a hierarchical medical speciality, administering the treatment. He/she may influence the patient by explaining their condition as a neurophysiological abnormality which has happened to them totally out of their control. New sophisticated techniques like magnetic resonance imaging (MRI) or positron emission tomography (PET) scanning and the dexamethasone suppression test (DST) tend to confirm this belief of a physical abnormality although the results are often inconclusive with only a certain percentage of patients in a particular category showing differences from 'normal' controls. This has led some researchers to hypothesise that biological indices are related to dimensions across categories and are not markers of illnesses.

Although all psychiatrists have a medical background, the disease model has been modified by the growth in specialities within the discipline such as liaison, transcultural and social psychiatry. These have led to a recognition of both the importance of other contributory factors in psychiatric disorders as well as to the influence of psychological factors on physical health.

The Psychodynamic Model

The psychodynamic model predates the biological movement in psychiatry, yet its founder, Freud, was from the discipline of neurology. Psychodynamic theory focuses on the mind or function of the brain in thought, feeling and behaviour and describes this function in its own language. The model is concerned with all aspects of the person. Freud described three levels of the self: the unconscious, primitive impulses of the id, the reason and common-sense of the ego and the self-criticism (via internalisation of parental figures) of the superego. The three systems are in constant interaction and psychiatric disorder is not seen as an illness but as a conflict between these different levels of functioning. Proponents do not believe that direct interviews elicit the important information as the conflict interferes in any interaction. However, the relationship between the therapist and patient (transference) is very important in elucidating and tackling this conflict. Symptoms are not accepted at face value but are indicative of mental conflict. There is no point in treating symptoms directly as they will reappear in another form (symptom substitution). Developmental aspects are very important as a person's early experiences and methods of coping with them have relevance to adult disorders. Bad experiences in childhood will inevitably affect later functioning although subsequent good relationships can ameliorate these to some extent. Psychodynamic theory is not solely concerned with psychiatric disorder and does not categorise patients, since conflict is present in everyone to a greater or lesser degree.

The Behavioural Model

The behavioural model developed from learning theory which has a scientific experimental basis in psychology. Psychological theory is founded in normal thinking and behaviour. Thus psychologists tend not to view psychiatric disorders as illnesses or categories but rather as an interaction between external events or stressors and personality. Personality is viewed as dimensional. Therefore the dimension of neuroticism investigated by Eysenck (1960) has a continuous distribution ranging from very stable and mature to unstable and immature. Someone at the unstable end would be much more likely to manifest symptoms. Symptoms are regarded as learned habits. When symptoms are distressing, they are described as maladaptive. Although the original learning is based on a very simple stimulus-response pairing various factors which reinforce responses or aid extinction have been isolated, and so it is known that maladaptive symptoms may generalise or persist because of avoidance. Treatment involves relearning and behavioural programmes to decrease maladaptive and increase adaptive behaviour are designed. Behavioural treatment usually takes the form of a contract between therapist and client. The contract sets out the goals of the treatment and methods of reaching them and the patient or client must be a willing participant in this scheme. Although the behavioural model has clear applications in certain psychiatric disorders e.g. phobias, more recently it has tended to be influenced by the recent emphasis on cognitive psychology and the intervening variables between the stimulus and response.

The Cognitive Model

The cognitive model is a relative newcomer to psychiatry. It developed from the dissatisfaction of both psychologists and psychiatrists with the behavioural and disease models' total disregard of the role of cognitive mechanisms in behaviour or illness and the purely theoretical formulations of psychoanalysis. It has thus influenced all these approaches. The cognitive model emphasises the role of cognitions (thoughts) within the interaction of thoughts, feelings and behaviour. The cognitive model of psychiatric disorders states that the patients' emotional response to an event is largely determined by the conscious meaning that is attributed to it. Significant events may activate or reinforce dysfunctional beliefs. The aims of treatment are first to identify these dysfunctional beliefs or assumptions; second to examine the relationship that occurs between negative thoughts resulting from them and both unpleasant emotions and maladaptive behaviour and third to challenge them against evidence and to correct them. The relationship between therapist and patient is a collaborative one. They work together to solve a problem by putting forward hypotheses and testing their validity. The cognitive model has had most influence in the treatment of depression but it is now being extended to other areas, often in an attempt to tackle symptoms not responsive to other forms of treatment.

The Social Model

The social model views society or social forces as most important in the development of psychiatric disorder. Durkheim's seminal work linked suicide to social disequilibrium or 'anomie' (Durkheim, 1987) and we now accept that isolation and alienation are predictive of depression. In addition, the impact of life events has been shown in all forms of psychiatric disorder. Symptoms and behaviour are considered in the social context in which they occur, thus relationships with other people are very important. Treatment aims to integrate the patient into an acceptable role within society again, usually by working on relationships. Thus marital (couple) therapy and family therapy are important developments. All the other models look to an internal explanation of a disorder but the social model reminds us that it is society which determines the boundary line between normal and abnormal behaviour. Behaviour which is acceptable in one society may not be in another and transcultural psychiatry has developed from this.

The Humanistic Model

The humanistic model emphasises important key qualities of the practitioner or therapist who is treating psychiatric disorders. These are empathy, warmth and understanding. Therapy may be termed 'client-centred' because the client is in control of what is discussed. The therapist helps the client to work out ways of dealing with problems by listening, asking questions, trying to understand and reflecting back (rephrasing what the client has said). More directive counselling may use additional interventions but requires similar non-judgemental therapist qualities. Simple intervention by a therapist with these qualities at an early stage may prevent a disorder developing and help the patient to mobilise their own coping skills and may be a reason for the growth in short-term therapies of all sorts. Patients seeking these qualities may account for the existence of numerous untested alternative therapies. The humanistic approach is a very powerful one and should be an important component of all therapies. It could be considered the epitome of good, clinical care.

The models described above are not mutually exclusive and in practice clinicians attempt to recognise the positive features of all models and use the most appropriate approach for each patient and set of circumstances. Certain models are associated with particular disorders and treatments. Thus, the psychoses are often linked to a biological approach requiring the use of psychotropic drugs, whereas the anxiety disorders may be understood by many in terms of learning theory requiring a behavioural approach. However, there is considerable overlap. The treatment of alcohol-related problems, for example, has been shown to include all the approaches outlined but whereas a few years ago the views of those advocating a disease or behavioural model were polarised, now there is evidence of integration of various treatment processes. Similarly, the approach to schizophrenia advocated by many specialists includes elements from several models (Figure 2.2). The practitioner often uses an eclectic approach intuitively, using various treatments with different patients or referring on to specialists in a particular method. However, it is important to remember that the treatment of psychiatric patients should be based on rigorous empirical study. The multiple factors leading to various disorders should be elucidated as well as the features of the disorder itself so that new effective treatments can be found.

THE PRINCIPLES OF PSYCHIATRIC DIAGNOSIS

Psychiatry is a branch of medicine and as such, much emphasis is placed on diagnosis. In general medicine, one diagnosis is usually sufficient and although psychiatry has attempted to refine its own diagnoses along the same lines multiple diagnoses or comorbidity are common. Diagnosis or classification has three main functions (Table 2.2). Firstly, it facilitates communication between clinicians and scientists both within the same area and across different countries and cultures. Secondly, it improves our knowledge about disorders, their probable course and pattern, i.e. prognosis. Thirdly, it helps us to decide on the appropriate treatment. In many branches of medicine, diagnosis of the problem or illness allows a precise definition and clearcut treatment but in illnesses in which knowledge is much less certain, like psychiatric disorders, the value and importance of diagnosis is correspondingly smaller.

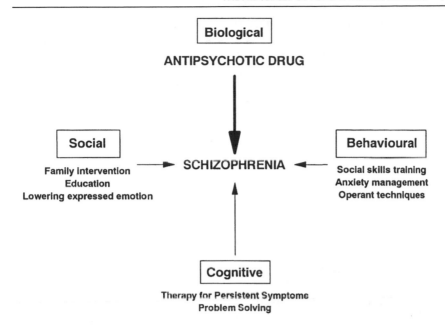

Figure 2.2   Treatment approach to schizophrenia incorporating several models

In psychiatry there are very few external criteria against which a diagnosis can be validated. Only the organic psychoses correspond to physical illnesses in the sense that objective evidence can be gained by a medical examination of the patient or from laboratory investigations. This means that the descriptive criteria upon which a psychiatric diagnosis is made need to be based on a consensus of clinicians and defined clearly. Equally, the conditions under which the diagnosis is made need to be carefully controlled. The information gathered from the patient should follow certain guidelines and the interview should be conducted in a standard way.

Over the past 30 years or so, the assessment of psychopathology in psychiatric conditions has been considerably improved. This has in large measure been due to the advances in the development of psychotropic drugs. The two fields of psychometrics in psychiatry and psychopharmacology have advanced hand in hand as drug companies seek indications for their newly

Table 2.2   Functions of diagnosis

Facilitation of communication
Information re: prognosis
Indications for treatment

developed treatments and existing treatments are found to aid apparently distinct conditions. The previous lack of a common classification system of psychiatric disorders defeated attempts at comparing different treatments and as the number of potentially effective treatments has increased, it has become more and more important to be able to compare them reliably in similar groups of patients. Much has already been achieved. There are now several standard diagnostic interviews (Table 2.3) based on the two major classification systems. The key features and time course of each disorder as well as other symptoms and signs are clearly defined and this has greatly improved agreement between assessors. These structured classification systems also use a multi-axial approach i.e. they take into account other important factors. Although clinical diagnosis is the primary factor, other factors such as personality, intellectual level, physical health and social circumstances are independently rated.

Method of Psychiatric Diagnosis

Diagnostic assessment in psychiatry is two-fold. The first stage is descriptive. Information from the referrer is combined with information gained from the patient at the interview to identify the presence (or absence) of a psychiatric disorder. This may be a matter of degree and reinforces the presence of a dimensional sphere if not instead at least in addition to the categorical. In fact many classification systems have scoring levels for symptoms depending on frequency and severity. The second stage of assessment is the construction of a working hypothesis (a 'formulation') about the nature of the disorder in which weight is assigned to the various factors, e.g. social, behavioural, physical symptoms, on which decisions about the treatment likely to be of most benefit to the individual are based. In major depressive disorder in which the patient complains of lack of sleep and appetite, it may be decided to institute drug treatment immediately, but if the primary complaint seems to be due to a poor marital relationship, it may be decided to try marital therapy.

Table 2.3   Main standardised diagnostic interviews based on classification systems

1. Schedule for Affective Disorders and Schizophrenia (SADS)	– based on RDC
2. Diagnostic Interview Schedule (DIS)	– based on RDC: DSM-III R
3. Structured Clinical Interview for DSM-III R (SCID)	– based on DSM-III R
4. Present State Examination (PSE)	– based on ICD-10: DSM-III R

RDC   Research Diagnostic Criteria
DSM   Diagnostic and Statistical Manual of Mental Disorders
ICD   International Classification of Diseases

Psychiatry and in particular the assessment of a disorder is a very inexact science. Using a classification system is an attempt to codify or standardise imprecise data but the procedures by which the information is gained are of equal concern. The initial interview is very important. The patient may be revealing intimate details about him/herself for the first time, and in order to do this must feel secure with the interviewer. On first acquaintance, the patient should be allowed to describe their problem freely as this shows the importance of various aspects of the problem to the individual concerned. A background history can then be obtained in which information not only about the development and course of the disorder but also genetic, social and personality factors is recorded. It is important that a diagnosis is not formed too quickly. There is evidence that the average psychiatric diagnosis is formed within two minutes of consultation and is seldom changed thereafter. There is therefore a danger that the interviewer's mind will close to other possibilities and new evidence at variance with the original diagnosis will at best not be sought or elicited and at worst, ignored. The clinician should always be open to new possibilities and should not rigidly adhere to a particular label. There may be wide variations between individuals awarded the same diagnosis or even within the same individual according to the stage of the disorder. This has led some professionals to advocate much broader categories, e.g. general neurotic syndrome.

Standard Diagnostic Interviews

A number of standard diagnostic interviews now exist based on the major classification systems (Table 2.3). The major difficulty for clinicians or researchers now lies in the choice of the best procedure for a particular use. They will not be described in detail here but a few examples will be outlined. The two major classification systems — Diagnostic and Statistical Manual of Mental Disorders (DSM) from the American Psychiatric Association (1994) and International Classification of Diseases (ICD) from the World Health Organisation (1992) — are constantly being refined and updated. Thus the Research Diagnostic Criteria (RDC) have largely been replaced by DSM-III, DSM-III R and now DSM-IV and similarly the ICD-8 is now ICD-10. Increasing international collaboration has meant that the two systems are converging in their descriptions of the major psychiatric disorders. Structured interviews are thus revised in light of the changes within both systems and some incorporate elements from both.

The Schedule for Affective Disorders and Schizophrenia (SADS) was designed to evaluate the symptoms of disorders as defined by the RDC. There are two main sections: the first dealing with the severity of patients' current conditions (mainly symptoms) defined by anchor points and the second covering the patients' lifetime history of psychiatric disorders prior to the year preceding the interview. The SADS procedure requires clinical psychiatric experience prior to specific training in administration. It is a time-consuming procedure (minimum one hour) but additional information from other sources may be used to aid clarification.

The Diagnostic Interview Schedule (DIS) is a fully structured diagnostic interview designed to be administered by non-clinicians originally in epidemiological research. Interviewers are trained in the procedure. Instead of clinical exploration of severity, a standard set of questions according to a probe flow chart is set out and this terminology should not be changed. The DIS takes a minimum of 40 mins to administer but the diagnosis is generated by computer, a very cost-effective procedure.

There has been considerable controversy over whether psychiatric diagnoses can be made by a fully structured survey instrument administered by non-clinicians. This led to the development of another clinician-administered interview: the Structured Clinical Interview for DSM-III R (SCID). Secondary aims were to produce an instrument superior to the SADS in training and administration time and in simplicity of diagnostic formulation from the gathered data. Thus the SCID is designed to assess diagnostic criteria rather than dimensional information on current status. Instead of six to seven points, there are three:

1. present and of clinically significant severity
2. present but of subthreshold severity
3. absent

Previous clinical experience and training are necessary.

The Present State Examination (PSE) was developed in the UK. It was intended as a clinical interview and the major focus is on symptomatology and functioning in the month prior to interview. Only information from the interview can be used to score items and the time limit of one month can make some diagnoses difficult to make. Interviewers are allowed to explore symptomatology in their own language and so clinical experience and training are necessary. There are numerous versions of the PSE, which is constantly being updated in line with the classification systems.

Although structured clinical interviews are sometimes used in studies evaluating psychotropic drug treatment, more often it is simply stated that patients meet the DSM-III R criteria or equivalent for a particular diagnosis. In many drug studies as well as those evaluating other forms of treatment no classification system is used, only severity scores on various rating scales.

THE HISTORY OF PSYCHOTROPIC DRUGS

The history of psychotropic drugs divides most easily into three eras (Figure 2.3). The first era begins with humans and their accidental discovery of plants with various mind altering qualities. Then from the middle of the 19th century simple organic chemicals like chloral began to be produced. The third and current phase began in the middle of this century with the synthesis and introduction of chlorpromazine, the discovery of the psychotropic effects of lithium, reserpine and the monoamine oxidase inhibitors. The changes in the present century must be set against other developments in psychiatry. The introduction of 'physical' methods of treatment like continuous narcosis, electroconvulsive therapy and leucotomy paved the way for the acceptance of drug treatment. In the same way, advances in other branches of pharmacology changed the attitudes of both the medical profession and the public towards drug treatment of psychiatric disorders.

Nevertheless, the history of psychopharmacology is largely serendipitous. Major advances were made unexpectedly and new drugs were found by chance. Thus although great progress has been made, it has been based much more on chance and the careful clinical observation of individual doctors who were prepared to experiment with various drugs to try and help their patients' psychiatric conditions than on any reliable method of scientific advancement.

Ancient Remedies

Alcohol is perhaps the best known psychotropic substance used right through the ages. It has been used therapeutically as an analgesic and anaesthetic and is still frequently used as an anxiolytic and an hypnotic. However its therapeutic value is outweighed by its social usage.

Opium, the solidified juice of the opium poppy, was cultivated even in prehistoric times. It was used, like alcohol, to lighten mood and to induce analgesia and sleep. Morphine was isolated from opium at the beginning of the 19th century and, during this century, the addictive properties of opium became increasingly apparent.

The resin of hemp — cannabis sativa — is known as hashish; the dried leaves and flowers of the same plant as marijuana. The intoxicating effects of this drug were known to people in ancient times and it was much used in the Islamic world of the Middle Ages. Despite its potential calming effects, it was not used therapeutically as part of medical practice.

There are many other drugs with psychotropic actions, too numerous to mention here. The discovery of new agents with similar properties has not

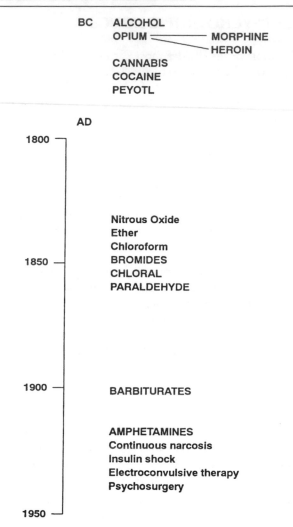

Figure 2.3   The history of psychotropic drugs and other physical treatments in psychiatry

meant the obsolescence of these ancient remedies, merely an extension of the alternative psychopharmacopeia.

Early Chemicals

The Industrial Revolution heralded the establishment of a chemical industry based on coal. Nitrous oxide was prepared in 1776 and its anaesthetic and euphoriant actions were recognised at the turn of the century but it was not until 50 years later that it was introduced as an anaesthetic. Ether and chloroform were used widely by this time.

In the mid-19th century bromides started to be used in the treatment of epilepsy. They rapidly became a panacea for all forms of psychiatric disorder despite their potential for poisoning. About the same time the hypnotic and anticonvulsant properties of chloral hydrate and paraldehyde were recognised. Chloral hydrate is still used but the most widely used of the early synthetic chemicals were the barbiturates. The first hypnotic barbiturate was introduced at the beginning of this century. A further 50 were marketed and some still survive although their use is now strictly limited because of the recognition of their dependence-producing potential and the discovery of much less toxic substances.

The amphetamines were synthesised in the late 1920s. They were found to combat fatigue and induce a sense of wellbeing in healthy individuals, leading to a wave of misuse. They were not, however, found to combat depression and so were not an advance in psychiatry.

The Development of Modern Psychotropic Drugs

Psychiatry had made considerable advances in the early 19th century. Classification of disorders had begun and the cruellest of treatment methods, including chaining, had been discontinued by the turn of the century. More tolerant public attitudes to those who were now considered mentally ill and the increasing emphasis on social measures of care and rehabilitation back into the community instead of incarceration in asylums gave impetus to the search for drug treatments. In 1899 Kraepelin's textbook on psychiatry included various drugs for the treatment of the mentally ill. Fifty years later the recommendations produced by Bleuler (1949) actually reduced the number of drugs, leaving out hashish and chloroform and cautioning against alcohol, and there were no new additions. It was against this background of reform that experimentation with modern psychotropic drugs began.

Chlorpromazine. Chlorpromazine was synthesised in the 1940s and a French surgeon (Laborit et al., 1952) experimenting with it in surgical shock, noticed the drug's unique capacity to induce tranquillisation without sedation and predicted its usefulness in psychiatry. Within a short time his prediction was confirmed and the medicine was recommended for a number of psychiatric conditions. Many other phenothiazines were synthesised and introduced and all proved to be valuable antipsychotic agents, alleviating delusions, hallucinations and disturbing behaviour, especially among schizophrenics.

Other antipsychotic drugs with slightly different structures, the thioxanthenes and butyrophenones, were developed not long afterwards. Reserpine, however, extracted from the rauwolfia serpentina plant, was found to be less effective than these new drugs.

Lithium. Lithium was discovered in the early 19th century and was used for a variety of conditions despite its known cardiotoxicity. In 1949 in Australia, Cade first pinpointed its antimanic action but for a variety of reasons it received little attention elsewhere in the world. This was partly because of its known toxicity, partly because mania is not a common complaint and partly because his discovery was overshadowed by the introduction of chlorpromazine. However, in the 1960s a Danish psychiatrist, (Schou, 1986) not only confirmed lithium's action on acute mania but also demonstrated its prophylactic effect in bipolar disorder. Thereupon, it again attracted interest and lithium clinics were set up for patients on chronic treatment.

Antidepressants. The first tricyclic antidepressant was imipramine. It was developed from a search for new antihistamines and was tried by a psychiatrist (Kuhn, 1958) in a few severely depressed patients. He was convinced of its efficacy and continued to use it in a series of such patients. He presented a detailed exposition of his observations confirming its antidepressant action. His description is a classic account and none of his claims of the clinical pattern of action of imipramine have since had to be significantly modified. The next tricyclic to be introduced was amitriptyline and although many others have since been marketed, none has proved to be more effective than these two.

The first MAOI antidepressant, iproniazid, was originally developed in 1959 as a medicament for the treatment of tuberculosis. It was noted to produce stimulant and euphoriant effects but initial trials in psychiatric patients were disappointing. A more systematic clinical investigation of its antidepressant effects was only commenced in 1956 after animal experiments had suggested it could prevent the sedating effects of reserpine. This indicated a biochemical rationale for the antidepressant action of iproniazid and it was much used in the USA. However, the toxicity of the drug soon became apparent, impeding further widespread use. It was withdrawn from the USA but remained on sale in some other countries including the UK. Other compounds like phenelzine and tranylcypromine were developed but the drugs were largely replaced by the tricyclics, their use being reserved for those failing to respond to other treatment.

Tranquillisers. The introduction of anxiolytic benzodiazepine drugs was not a novel advance in the same way as chlorpromazine or imipramine. These drugs closely resemble alcohol and the barbiturates. The use of the sedatives, however, was severely restricted by their narrow therapeutic range and the risk of habituation and dependence. The first link in the chain to benzodiazepines was forged by the discovery of mephenesin, a muscle relaxant with anxiolytic properties. This drug was too short-acting to be of any clinical use but eventually meprobamate was developed and enjoyed extensive use and commercial success until the introduction of the benzodiazepines. Work on these drugs began as part of Hoffman-La Roche's decision to support planned pharmacological testing in known experimental settings. Sternbach, a chemist, chose to work again on a class of substances he had first synthesised in the 1930s in Cracow (Sternbach, 1978). Most of these substances proved to be pharmacologically uninteresting but one, chlordiazepoxide, was found to have hypnotic, sedative and anticonvulsant properties. The first clinical tests nearly led to it being discarded because too large a dose was given to geriatric patients, causing ataxia and dysarthria. However, lower doses established its clinical effectiveness and its congener, diazepam, proved to be even more successful.

Future Developments. The prototypes of modern psychotropic drugs were discovered in a period of about 10 years (Figure 2.4). Neither before nor since has such a series of clinical advances been made in psychopharmacology. These discoveries did not follow a common pattern and few were targeted, i.e. developed with a specific therapeutic indication in mind. They did, however, lead to extensive study of drug mechanisms, brain chemistry and biological aspects of psychiatry. However, we should be aware that theories based on existing partially effective psychotropic solutions are unlikely to lead to, and may actually prevent, totally new discoveries.

The Classification of Psychotropic Drugs

A vast number of chemical agents affect the behaviour and mental processes of humans. However, in this book, we are only concerned with those which are used therapeutically in psychiatry. Other substances with a psychotropic or psychoactive action such as alcohol, nicotine, cocaine and heroin only concern us insofar as dependence on them can be treated. Drugs used to treat physical illnesses but which also have some psychotropic action will only be considered if they have a therapeutic role in psychiatry e.g. beta-blockers, antihistamines.

Psychotropic drugs can be classified in various ways e.g. according to their chemical structure, their biological actions or their main therapeutic indications. An early attempt in 1931 to classify them according to their actions on mental processes produced five independent categories:

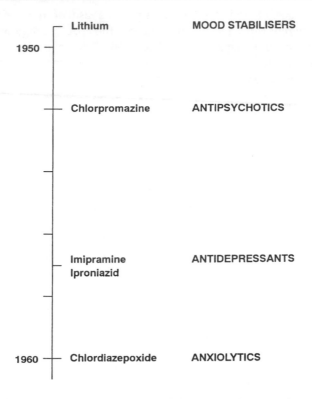

Figure 2.4   The chronological development of prototypes of modern psychotropic drugs

euphoriants; phantastica; inebriantia; hypnotica and excitantia. This was way ahead of contemporary thinking and probably the forerunner of our current system as other classification systems used until the advent of chlorpromazine merely divided psychotropics into two categories: depressants and stimulants.

The major advances in psychopharmacology in the 1950s meant this division was inadequate and led to the naming of these new groups of drugs mainly by clinicians, e.g. major and minor tranquillisers. The terms proved difficult to define and were attacked by pharmacologists. However, efforts to identify the key pharmacological actions of psychotropic drugs have proved difficult because most of the drugs are pharmacologically 'dirty' i.e. they have multiple actions. Efforts to produce 'cleaner' drugs have improved side-effect profiles rather than therapeutic action and it may be that a particular combination of pharmacological actions is necessary to combat various features of a psychiatric disorder. The classification system which has resulted and which has received common agreement (Table 2.4) is a combination of old terms, hypnotics, new terms, anxiolytics and descriptive terms, antipsychotics. Within each broad classification, which is generally based on clinical action, the subclassification often refers to the chemical nature or action of the compound, monoamine oxidase inhibitor (MAOI) or selective serotonin reuptake inhibitor (SSRI), which is thought to be relevant to the primary indication. Another group of drugs which used to be included in the table was hallucinogens, e.g. LSD. However, despite their profound effects on mental processes, these have been found to have no therapeutic action and so will not be discussed further.

The antipsychotics are also referred to as the neuroleptics. Their primary indication is the treatment of schizophrenia and other psychotic states. There are numerous chemical subtypes which mainly differ in their side-effect profile

Table 2.4   A current classification system of psychotropic drugs

Major drug groups	Main indication
ANTIPSYCHOTICS	
Phenothiazines	Schizophrenia
Thioxanthenes	
Dibenzapines	
Indoles	
Butyrophenones	
Diphenylpiperidines	
ANTIDEPRESSANTS	
Tricyclics	Depression
Monoamine oxidase inhibitors	
Selective serotonin reuptake inhibitors	
Reversible inhibitors of monoamine oxidase	
MOOD STABILISERS	
Lithium	Mania
	Bipolar disorder
ANXIOLYTICS	
Benzodiazepines	Anxiety
Azapirones	
HYPNOTICS	
Benzodiazepines	Sleep
Cyclopyrrolones	
Imidazopyrimidines	
STIMULANTS	Minimal brain dysfunction
APPETITE SUPPRESSANTS	Obesity
NOOTROPICS	Dementia

rather than their therapeutic action. The antidepressants are mainly used to treat depression. There are various subgroups with different pharmacological actions but again the difference is greater with respect to side-effects than efficacy. Mood-stabilising drugs include lithium, valproate and carbamazepine. Lithium has a specific anti-manic action and can be used prophylactically in bipolar disorder. Its potential for cardiotoxicity and narrow therapeutic range have led to its decreased use at various times but lower doses and careful monitoring of blood levels and adverse effects have minimised such risks. The anxiolytics used to be referred to as sedatives, then minor tranquillisers. The change in name partly reflects the increased specificity. Many drugs are sedative without particularly helping anxiety. The benzodiazepines are still the main drugs in this class but there has been an attempt to make them more specific and less dependence-inducing by reducing their agonist effect on gamma-aminobutyric acid (GABA). A newer class of anxiolytic with a totally different pharmacology are the azapirones. The benzodiazepines are also the main class of hypnotics but older drugs like chloral are sometimes used and newer ones like zopiclone and zolpidem have recently been introduced.

There are various other classes of psychotropic drugs with limited indications. The stimulants used to be widely used to combat fatigue, improve performance and suppress appetite but because of their potential for dependence and abuse, their use is now controlled. They are now only indicated in children for the treatment of hyperactivity or attention deficit disorder in which they have a paradoxical effect. They are used widely in the USA but are still uncommon in Europe. Newer classes of appetite suppressant are more specific with little stimulant or euphoriant action and therefore insignificant abuse potential. Nootropic drugs have been developed in an attempt to halt the progressive decline of dementia. They are intended to have a beneficial effect on cognition without inducing general stimulation.

Although each of the major drug groups has a main indication, they also have therapeutic effects on other disorders. One drug may be beneficial in several disorders e.g. SSRIs are not only effective in depression but also help eating disorders and obsessive-compulsive disorder. Attempts have therefore been made to show that these disorders are rooted in depression but the drugs may also help the primary complaint when there is no evidence of depression; there are many other examples of a drug being effective in many disorders. This may be because psychotropic drugs generally have multiple actions and even those which are claimed to be specific to one neurotransmitter, also indirectly influence others. In the same way, one disorder may be improved by many different treatments. Depression may be improved by TCAs, SSRIs, antipsychotics, ECT as well as psychological treatments. This may indicate that depression is a multifaceted condition and different aspects respond to different approaches or it may reflect the rather low level of sophistication of our current systems of classification within psychiatry. It is important, however, that we continue to try to improve these systems and seek new methods of treatment. As we have seen, really original discoveries have often been based more on the strong clinical motivation of individual researchers than any newly acquired basic knowledge.

SUMMARY

Different models of psychiatric disorder are often associated with particular disorders or treatments. Increasingly a multidisciplinary approach is being used, recognising the value of different treatments for various aspects of a disorder. Psychiatric diagnosis is an imprecise science but there are various techniques that can help to standardise clinical judgement. Although mind-altering substances have been used since ancient times, the major developments in psychopharmacology occurred around the 1950s when all the major groups of psychotropic drugs were discovered. More recent developments are based on refinements of these. Psychotropic drugs are generally classified according to their main indication.

FURTHER READING

American Psychiatric Association (1994) *Diagnostic and Statistical Manual of Mental Disorders* (4th revised edn). American Psychiatric Press, Washington, D.C.

Beck, A.T. (1966) *Depression*. University of Pennsylvania Press, Philadelphia.

Bleuler, E. (1949) *Lehrbuch der Psychiatrie* (8th edn). Springer, Berlin.

Brown, J.A.C. (1961) *Freud and the Post-Freudians*. Penguin, London.

Cade, J.F. (1949) Lithium salts in the treatment of psychotic excitement. *Medical Journal of Australia* **2**, 349–352.

Durkheim, E. (1987) *Le Suicide*. Translated 1952 as *Suicide: A Study in Sociology* (Spaulding, J.A. and Simpson, G., eds). Routledge and Kegan Paul, London.

Ellis, A. (1962) *Reason and Emotion in Psychotherapy*. Lyle Stuart, New York.

Eysenck, H.J. (ed.) (1960) *Handbook of Abnormal Psychology*. Pitman, London.

Freeman, H.L. (ed.) (1984) *Mental Health and the Environment*. Churchill Livingstone, London.

Kraepelin, E., (1899) *Psychiatrie. Ein Lehrbuch für Studirende und Aerzte* (6th edn). J.A. Barth, Leipzig.

Kuhn, R. (1958) The treatment of depressive states with G22355 (imipramine hydrochloride). *American Journal of Psychiatry*, **115**, 459–463.

Laborit, H., Huguenard, P. and Alluaume, R. (1952) Un nouveau stabilisateur végétatif (le 4560 R.P.). *Presse Med.* **60**, 206–208.

Morgenstern, J. and McCrady, B.S. (1992) Curative factors in alcohol and drug treatment: behavioural and disease model perspectives. *British Journal of Addiction* **87**, 901–912.

Pichot, P. (1994) Nosological models in psychiatry. *British Journal of Psychiatry* **164**, 232–240.

Robertson, M.M. (1989) The assessment of mood and its components. In *Human Psychopharmacology: Measures and Methods*, vol. 2 (Hindmarch, I. and Stonier, P.D., eds). John Wiley, Chichester, pp. 67–126.

Rogers, K. (1951) *Client-Centered Therapy: Its Current Practice, Implications and Theory*. Houghton Mifflin, Boston.

Sartorius, N., de Girolamo, G., Andrews, G., German, G.A. and Eisenberg, L. (eds) *Treatment of Mental Disorders*. World Health Organisation Publication. American Psychiatric Press, Washington, D.C.

Schou, M. (1986) Lithium treatment: a refresher course. *British Journal of Psychiatry* **149**, 541–547.

Sternbach, L. (1978) The benzodiazepine story. In *Progress in Drug Research*, vol. 22 (Jucker, E., ed.). Birkhäuser, Basle, pp. 229–266.

Thompson, C. (ed.) (1989) *The Instruments of Psychiatric Research*. John Wiley, Chichester.

Tyrer, P. and Steinberg, D. (1993) *Models for Mental Disorder. Conceptual Models in Psychiatry*, (2nd edn). John Wiley, Chichester.

World Health Organisation (1992) *The International Classification of Mental and Behavioural Disorders*. World Health Organisation, Geneva.

Chapter 3

SOCIAL AND PSYCHOLOGICAL ASPECTS OF DRUG TREATMENT

In this chapter we discuss the non-pharmacological aspects of drug treatment such as the factors influencing doctors to prescribe and patients' attitudes towards drug treatment. Non-compliance may lead to mistaken assumptions about treatment inefficacy and so ways of improving compliance are outlined. The characteristics of psychological and physical dependence are described and the importance of the placebo effect in any treatment is acknowledged.

DRUG PRESCRIBING

In pharmacology, drugs are chemicals which alter physiological functions. However, once they are prescribed, they exist in a social context and they have psychological effects as well. The decision to prescribe a drug is not based solely on medical grounds but is also a reaction to a social situation. Psychotropic drugs are prescribed to alter psychological functioning and are therefore even more subject to these effects. When faced with a patient's emotional distress, a doctor is likely to respond by offering a prescription. However, doctors in the UK have been shown to prescribe more rationally than those in Italy, Germany or France. Their decisions are more likely to be based on proven drug efficacy and they avoid using ineffective drugs or several drugs simultaneously (polypharmacy).

Pattern of Prescribing

The advent of the new psychotropic drugs earlier this century led to major changes in the treatment of and attitudes towards people with psychiatric disorders. This was largely beneficial. It allowed patients who had previously led very restricted lives because of their problems and disabilities, a chance to reintegrate into society. However, emotional distress and psychological symptoms are very common and there has been a steady growth in prescriptions so that now 1 person in 10 of the British population is prescribed a psychotropic drug during any one year. Much of this use is short-term and about half of the patients who start treatment will have stopped within a month.

Until recently, when new psychotropic agents were introduced, their use tended to be initially in the hands of psychiatrists. However, as their safety and efficacy became established, they were prescribed more and more often by those without psychiatric or psychopharmacological expertise. This often had major social implications. Nowadays, the major prescribers of psychotropic drugs are GPs, often from the start, and about 15% of all prescriptions written by GPs are for these drugs. The most commonly prescribed are benzodiazepines as night-time hypnotics and to a lesser extent as daytime anxiolytics. Prescriptions for benzodiazepines rose steadily during the 1960s and 1970s but as the risk of dependence with chronic use became recognised, the total number started to decline in the 1980s. In six years (1979–1985) it declined by 16% and there has been a further decline to 18 million scripts in 1990 (23% of the 1985 figure). It is now known that the rate of prescribing of anxiolytics has declined more rapidly than that of hypnotics which has hardly altered.

Studies examining the characteristics of benzodiazepine use have isolated certain key factors (Table 3.1). Factors such as psychological malaise and elevated neuroticism seem easy to explain as benzodiazepines are largely prescribed for anxiety. Other social factors such as gender, age, socio-economic status and unemployment have been explained as social control of powerless groups in society. However, all types of prescribing are increased in unemployed people perhaps because of associated poverty and morbidity and may represent an attempt by the GP to improve the tolerability of life of the most disadvantaged groups in society. A study of medical students showed that they were more willing to engage in helping behaviour (prescribing medication) when patients' life events were regarded as

Table 3.1   Factors associated with current benzodiazepine use

Female gender
Increased age
Physical ill-health
Psychological malaise
Elevated neuroticism scores
Lower socio-economic status
Unemployment
Current smoking
Less participation in active leisure pursuits

uncontrollable rather than controllable. Increased prescribing to women has been explained by their stressful role in society, their increased use of medical facilities and their willingness to talk about emotional problems. Some confirmation is given to this by the fact that women are also more frequently referred to counselling services within the NHS and this is often for relationship problems.

Factors Influencing Doctors to Prescribe

Although we do not know why some doctors prescribe more than others, certain factors are known to influence the decision to prescribe (Table 3.2).

Peer Communication

Education is a continuing process for prescribers as new drugs are licensed and promoted. Information comes not only from reports of clinical trials of both new drug and non-drug treatments, but from communications from hospital consultants. Although GPs may learn of new treatments in this way, studies have shown that consultants often fail to give important information or to make clear which doctor has clinical responsibility and therefore responsibility for prescribing. GPs may feel they have inadequate expertise in administering new treatments and may feel particularly concerned about the information they are now expected to give to patients. More informal peer contact may provide more relevant information. It has been shown that GPs with membership of a local medical network and frequent social contacts with peers will try a new drug before GPs who are more isolated.

The Pharmaceutical Industry

Doctors gain most of their information about new drugs from the pharmaceutical industry. Modern advertising is carefully constructed to fulfil the desires of the consumer. An image is built up to appeal to the target consumer, in this case the prescriber. Selecting the product is portrayed as making treatment easy. Before prescribing, a doctor has many decisions to

Table 3.2 Factors influencing doctors to prescribe

Peer communication — formal and informal
Advertising
Patient expectation and demand
Existence and knowledge of alternatives

make: Is it necessary? What will it achieve? Which is the best treatment? Does the benefit outweigh the harm? The advert may affect their judgement on each point. Scientific evidence in the form of references is often provided to confirm the claims but most adverts are only given a quick glance; so impressions are more important than facts. Apart from advertisements, many doctors also receive visits from representatives of drug companies. Although GPs are reluctant to admit that representatives influence their prescribing decisions and are increasingly reluctant to devote much time to them, they can be the first source of knowledge about new products and are helpful for reporting any adverse reactions. In the rapidly changing field of medicine, representatives are likely to provide a readily available and easily accessible form of continuing education.

Patient Expectations/Demands

GPs are influenced by their patients' expectations about treatment and their anxiety about their health. Patients expecting a prescription are five times more likely to receive one and patients who are anxious about their health problems are 50% more likely to receive a prescription irrespective of their expectations. A number of patients in mental distress do not put forward that need to their GP when they visit but present only physical problems. Anxiety about these may lead the GP to suspect a psychological disorder.

Existence and Knowledge about Alternatives

The existence of alternative, available methods of treating psychological distress may decrease the amount of prescribing especially for minor disorders. Thus a recent study examining GPs' views on the treatment of anxiety found most agreed that counselling could be as effective as benzodiazepines. They felt it was too demanding of their own time but two-thirds were in favour of employing counsellors in their practice and over 50% favoured the increased availability of clinical psychology services. Knowledge of other organisations such as self-help groups may also decrease prescribing.

Factors Influencing Patient Views Towards Prescribing

Drug use is part of illness and health behaviour. There is evidence that patients are now less happy to receive a prescription at the end of a consultation. They appear to have changed their attitudes faster than doctors in realising that psychotropic drugs are not always appropriate, especially where the cause seems to be mainly psychosocial. In fact most people tolerate their symptoms for some time before they consult their GP. They often try alternative solutions first and such self-help can be very effective. When patients do consult their GP, they are likely to have expectations of treatment based on how they think doctors in general would respond to a patient's emotional distress. These views are likely to have been influenced by three factors: the impact of psychiatric notions on lay thinking; the influence of the media; and the impact of their own direct experience of using services or taking psychotropic drugs. The last is the most salient but expectations of it come from the first two. Patients' experiences of psychiatric treatment differ from those of other medical services largely because of stigma.

Impact of Psychiatric Notions

Psychiatry has had far greater legitimation problems in promoting a persuasive ideology than other medical specialities. It has had problems establishing itself within medicine. Traditionally psychiatric services were isolated from other medical facilities in remote psychiatric hospitals. This led to alienation but the change to liaison psychiatry and community care has improved the situation. The medical model of psychiatric disorder has also had to contend with the growth and credibility of the alternative models of psychiatric disorder. Probably the model most familiar to the general public is the psychoanalytic one, which bears little relationship to standard psychiatric practice and tends to be anti drug treatment.

Influence of the Media

The media are a powerful influence on views towards psychiatric disorder and its treatment. They assume a role of both educating the public about possible biological causes and potential new drug treatments while at the same time producing sensational accounts of potential negative effects. This has been seen recently with both triazolam and fluoxetine. It is rare to find a balanced, informed approach as reporters prefer to opt for the sensational story. However, it is often the first source to alert the public to new drugs or alternative types of treatment, thus promoting patient choice and self-help.

Patient Experiences

It might be expected that users of psychiatric services would have more positive views towards treatment than the general population. In confirmation of this, anxious patients attending a psychiatric out-patient clinic have been shown to have generally more positive attitudes towards their doctor, medicine and hospital care than matched healthy controls. However, few studies have looked at patient views towards different types of treatment. One recent study interviewed 516 psychiatric patients who had had at least one psychiatric admission to hospital. Attitudes to drug treatments were dependent not only on the actual drugs involved but also on administration. Antidepressants were seen in a favourable light by most users because their use was oral and voluntary. However, attitudes to antipsychotics depended on the attitude of the prescriber and whether use was compulsory. Although 57% rated them as helpful, their use in rapid tranquillisation was often seen as punitive, particularly if it was associated with other restrictive measures such as withdrawal of privileges, seclusion or lack of care from staff. It is interesting that similar attitudes were expressed about ECT: it could be helpful but was frightening especially if administered without consent. It is very important that health professionals explain treatments and negotiate a treatment plan to reduce anxiety. Non-physical treatments like occupational and industrial therapy were viewed as helpful by 58% and 61% of the patients respectively but differences in satisfaction were related to the perceived attitudes of psychiatrists and the flexibility and relevance of the scheme to the individual. Counselling and psychotherapy received the most positive assessment (74%) and this was unrelated to other factors such as psychiatrist attitude. Satisfaction was related to length of contact (>5 sessions) and being informed of the therapeutic approach. Patients valued the chance of being listened to and understood as an individual. Patients are more likely to comply with treatments which they view as helpful.

TREATMENT COMPLIANCE

Compliance is an important factor in any treatment procedure and non-compliance may lead to mistaken assumptions about treatment inefficacy. However the consequences of non-compliance are potentially more dangerous with drug treatment. Failing to take an antibiotic correctly may lead to a worsening of a respiratory infection and even hospitalisation. Taking a barbiturate at inappropriately short intervals may lead to unintentional overdose. Failing to adhere to the dietary restrictions while taking an MAOI may lead to a severe hypertensive crisis. The potential consequences are even worse when multiple drugs are being taken. Non-compliance may be deliberate or unintentional. In general it is undesirable but sometimes it can be beneficial e.g. if a patient develops an intolerable adverse reaction and discontinues treatment immediately, or if the wrong drug is dispensed and the patient recognises the error. Therefore the patient's reasons for non-compliance should always be examined.

Non-compliance with prescribed drugs can take two forms: the prescription may never be dispensed or if it is dispensed, the drug may not be taken as directed. These have been termed primary and secondary. The rate of primary non-compliance has been estimated to be about 20%. Secondary non-compliance may take several forms. The patient may take no drugs at all, too few, too many, at the wrong time of day and so on. The rate of secondary non-compliance is higher (15%–90%) and much more difficult to measure. Various methods have been used from pill counts, canister weighing, bottle caps which record usage to plasma concentrations, but none is ideal to measure all aspects of drug-taking and none is foolproof.

Determinants of Compliance

Certain factors have been shown to be important in compliance (Table 3.3).

Demographic Factors

Men and women are equally likely to be poor compliers. However, non-compliance is associated with younger age, poor socio-economic background and social isolation. The patient's perception of financial distress, whether real or imaginary, tends to lead to non-compliance even when medication is free.

Drug Variables

The way in which a drug has to be taken influences compliance. Thus, once-a-day formulations aid compliance compared with more frequent dosing. Drugs with no obvious benefit to the recipient, such as antihypertensives, or with a delayed therapeutic effect, such as antidepressants, present problems with compliance. However, the most important drug factor in compliance is adverse effects. Dysphoria experienced shortly after administration is a predictor of poor compliance. Other adverse reactions leading to poorer quality of life, e.g. interference in sleep, sexual dysfunction, excessive sedation, also reduce compliance. Sometimes patients may self-regulate their medication by changing the time or dose to avoid such effects and have more control over their lives. In the case of more severe side-effects such as with

Table 3.3 Determinants of compliance

Demographic factors
Drug variables
Patient characteristics
Treatment setting
Doctor–patient relationship
Practical considerations

antipsychotics, clinicians are often reluctant to inform patients fully about possible adverse reactions because of worries about compliance. However this could be held to be a breach of duty of care which, if it causes the patient injury, might render the doctor liable to a claim for compensation. In the past, English law has tended to side with the doctor but public opinion is changing in accordance with other countries to take the patient's perspective into account. Manufacturers' patient information leaflets are now legally required for all newly licensed prescription medicines, helping to inform the patient of potential risks but these are not intended to absolve the doctor from responsibility.

Patient Variables

Good compliance is associated with the patient's perception of his/her condition and the estimated success of any intervention. The ability to understand and retain information given are important factors. On average 60% of oral information is forgotten. Negative attitudes to drug treatment inevitably decrease compliance but studies have found it impossible to discriminate between partial and wholly compliant patients. The fear of becoming dependent on a psychotropic drug is an important factor in both primary and secondary compliance. The need for continuation of prophylactic treatment may not be understood. Lack of insight or denial of a psychiatric condition leads both to primary non-compliance and forms of secondary non-compliance like stopping medication prematurely. However, it is important not to interpret non-compliance as automatically meaning lack of insight. The patient is also affected by family attitudes to drugs and expectations of outcome.

Treatment Setting

Compliance rates are often measured in research settings but these clearly differ from the usual clinical settings. In research studies, the frequency and spacing of visits is specified, the patient usually sees the same clinician and patients are often followed up if they do not attend. These all encourage compliance but the fact that the treatment is assigned in a random and double-blind fashion and the patient may have to travel to the centre may do the reverse. Different factors therefore need to be taken into account when considering compliance in different treatment settings.

Doctor–patient Relationship

The concept of compliance can be seen to be paternalistic. It assumes the doctor knows best and the patient cannot make a contrary decision. Some researchers have therefore suggested changing the term to 'adherence' but changing a name does not in itself change the interaction. Thus compliance is dependent on the relationship between doctor and patient in terms of quality, duration and frequency of interaction. Both the doctor's attitude to the patient and the information given are of prime importance.

Practical Considerations

It is important not to neglect certain practical matters which may interfere with compliance. The patient may have difficulty picking up the prescription, or the pharmacist may not have the drug in stock. There may be a change of doctors or residence. Intercurrent illnesses or prearranged events may make compliance impossible or unlikely. All these factors should be considered in examining compliance rates.

Improving Patient Compliance

Various approaches to the management of non-compliance have been used. The three major methods involve education, behavioural techniques and increasing collaboration (Table 3.4)

Education

In order to both derive benefit and avoid harm from psychotropic drugs, patients need certain information. The mandatory inclusion of information leaflets has helped this but should not be a substitute for doctors giving oral and other written information about how and when to take the medicine, precautions and interactions. It is easy for doctors to overestimate the ability of patients to understand technical terms which are familiar to them e.g. hypertension, sublingual. It is especially important that the doctor states the purposes of treatment as some drugs are given for many conditions and dose may vary according to indication. The prescriber should also warn of stopping drugs abruptly. Although some doctors are wary of giving full information about side-effects, studies addressing this question have found that informing patients about side-effects reduced their anxiety about

Table 3.4   Improving patient compliance

Psychoeducation procedures
Behavioural approaches
Creating a therapeutic alliance

treatment without adversely affecting compliance. It is important to balance information about the drug with information about the condition and possible ways of treating it. Where lack of insight or poor comprehension are likely to impede compliance, it is often helpful to involve relatives in the education process. Psychoeducation or formal teaching programmes, including information about both condition, medication and the importance of adhering to a certain regimen, has been shown to improve compliance.

Behavioural Interventions

Two types of behavioural interventions have been evaluated: a skills-based approach and the use of cues and monitoring. The skills-based approach provides similar information to the education approach but uses techniques such as role-play, overlearning and modelling to reinforce learning. Monitoring of pill-taking via electronic devices and giving feedback helps patients understand their pattern of drug usage and improves compliance. Although both these approaches have been shown to increase patient compliance, a major drawback is that they rely to some extent on the patient's compliance with the programme. They are thus only likely to have an effect on secondary rather than primary non-compliance.

Therapeutic Alliance

The third approach is to attempt to strengthen the doctor-patient relationship by creating a therapeutic alliance. Much weight is given to this in therapeutic models of psychiatric disorder. It is an essential component in all except the biological model. There appears to be a tendency for patients to show greater compliance with psychological as opposed to drug treatment regimens, probably because of the emphasis on collaboration. However it is still a relevant issue and a negative attitude to the therapist and unwillingness to engage in self-exploration have been shown to correlate with non-compliance with cognitive behavioural therapy. In drug treatment it has been shown that patients who establish an appropriate therapeutic alliance, are not only more compliant with medication but need less of it and have a better clinical outcome. The provision of supportive psychotherapy has been shown to lead to a lower probability of relapse once medication is withdrawn. The important factors seem to be patient choice and a negotiated treatment plan which has certain requirements (Table 3.5). All the options should be explained to the patient and the treatment plan should be jointly agreed. Motivational interviewing is one example of this approach. The clinician focuses on specific costs and benefits of the treatment regimen but encourages the patient to take responsibility for making the decisions.

Table 3.5   Ways to enhance compliance via the therapeutic relationship

— Listen to the patient
— Give information about the condition
— Acknowledge possible stigma
— Understand the patient's goals and expectations
— Describe treatment options
— Explain risks and benefits of treatment
— Involve the patient in the decision

DRUG DEPENDENCE AND WITHDRAWAL

Dependence

Drug dependence is characterised by a compulsion to take a drug either to experience psychic effects or to avoid the physical or psychological discomfort of its absence. However misuse is not a prerequisite for dependence to occur as therapeutically prescribed drugs, taken according to instructions, may cause both physical and psychological dependence. Psychotropic drugs are taken for their effects on the psyche and so it is difficult to decide whether the compulsion to take the drug is a consequence of addiction or therapeutic need.

Stopping any treatment may lead to a recurrence of the original symptoms of the disorder or to an increase in non-specific symptoms because of psychological dependence resulting in a desire to reinstitute that treatment whether it was a benzodiazepine, an antidepressant or psychotherapy. Stopping a drug may also lead to withdrawal symptoms. Although these are signs typical of the physiological systems originally modified by the drug (rebound hyperexcitability) they are new to the patient and this is known as physiological dependence. The severity of withdrawal symptoms varies with the degree of dependence. Thus it has been suggested that rebound anxiety a few hours after a drinking bout or the typical hangover the morning after drinking a significant amount of alcohol is on a continuum with the experience of severe alcohol withdrawal symptoms after many years of very heavy intake.

Psychological dependence may occur without evidence of physical dependence but psychotropic drug intake usually results in a combination of the two. Certain characteristics of both the substance and the consumer are important.

Properties of Substance

Drug preference studies show us a substance's potential for abuse but do not mean dependence or abuse are inevitable. Neither does the absence of preference or liking automatically exclude abuse. Certain properties of a drug and its administration make dependence more likely.

Reinforcement. A drug is reinforcing if it has effects which the user likes and desires to re-experience, e.g. euphoria.

Dose. Higher doses are likely to lead to more marked effects on withdrawal. Severe reactions are more common with doses above the recommended therapeutic range.

Rapid action. Rapid absorption and penetration to the brain mean the drug has the desired effect very quickly. Other pharmacokinetic variables such as high oral bioavailability, low protein binding and a small volume of distribution also mean that higher concentrations of the drug are reached in the bloodstream (see Chapter 4).

Elimination rate. A drug which has a short half-life or which has a high free drug clearance and so is metabolised and cleared quickly is likely to result in an earlier and more severe rebound effect. The user is also more likely to relate these effects to drug use because of the timing.

Regular intake. Regular rather than intermittent use leads to a greater likelihood of dependence. A cigar at Christmas is unlikely to lead to nicotine dependence.

Length of administration. The longer a drug is taken, the more likely it is to cause dependence. However after a certain period of continuous use, it may make no difference.

Rate of termination. Abrupt termination is more likely to lead to severe withdrawal symptoms. Gradual withdrawal or substance substitution will reduce the effect.

Tolerance. Tolerance can be defined as the reduced effect of the same dose of a drug on subsequent administrations which results in a need to increase the dose in order to maintain the same level of effect. It is common with certain drugs of abuse e.g. LSD, heroin. It used to be thought that tolerance was a necessary prerequisite to dependence. However tolerance is a complicated phenomenon. It may occur at different rates to various properties of the drug and the extent of tolerance differs both within and between drugs for a given subject. It is therefore difficult to predict reliably and certainly full tolerance is not necessary for dependence to occur.

Characteristics of Person

The characteristics of a person who is likely to become dependent on a substance are difficult to evaluate. However a few indicators have been found.

Biological factors. People show marked individual differences in their potential to become dependent on drugs. There seems to be a genetic factor in the development of alcohol-related problems.

Age. The age at which a drug is first ingested seems to be important for dependence on nicotine, and drug abuse or experimentation is more common among the young.

Previous experience. A person who has shown previous dependence on other drugs or treatments is more likely to become dependent on a new substance. It is important to be aware of this when, for example, treating alcohol-related problems with benzodiazepines.

Multiple drugs. The more drugs which are taken simultaneously, the more likely dependence is to occur on at least one of them.

Personality. Certain personality characteristics have been identified as indicating a risk for dependence. People who score higher on measures of neuroticism or passive-dependent personality and who have fewer methods of coping leading to less resourcefulness are more at risk. Thus people prescribed benzodiazepines for a psychiatric condition are more likely to become dependent than those prescribed them for a medical condition. Social and environmental factors are also important. Thus although alcohol is generally seen as a social enhancer, large quantities may be taken to mask anxiety and social isolation. Peer group pressure is very relevant in the consumption of nicotine and illicit drugs.

Withdrawal

At one time it was thought that the presence of a withdrawal syndrome determined drug dependence. Now it is seen as a contributory factor. Withdrawal syndromes have been delineated for many drugs. The opioid withdrawal syndrome has been the longest studied and the best described. It has been described as a flu-like illness with muscle aching and gastric disturbance, more apparent to the sufferer than the observer. Craving is a key feature preceding physical discomfort and leading to drug-seeking behaviour. Withdrawal from alcohol and benzodiazepines is also associated with somatic symptoms like sweating and tremor and can involve perceptual disturbances. The nicotine withdrawal syndrome consists of physiological changes such as decreased adrenaline, cortisol, and heart-rate, weight gain and increased taste for sweets. Numerous psychological changes have been reported e.g. increased irritability, anxiety and sleep disturbance. Some of the signs and symptoms of the various drug withdrawal syndromes overlap. Certainly mood disturbance is a key feature in all of them but it is difficult to establish whether this is due to pharmacological effects or psychological processes. Stopping any drug may therefore lead to psychological problems and this is partly due to the placebo effect.

THE PLACEBO EFFECT

Any treatment embodies certain psychological components which may be described as 'the placebo effect'. With a drug, these are effects over and above its chemical properties. Although placebo effects are non-specific, they are not therapeutically inactive and their effectiveness compared to no treatment is often ignored. Placebo effects are therefore important in the evaluation of all interventions, not just drug treatment, but this has often been neglected in determining the efficacy of psychological treatments. Because psychological factors are so important in the success of a particular intervention, some authors have argued for maximising any non-specific placebo effects clinically. The placebo effect has been found to be affected by various factors.

Type of placebo. Much has been written about the physical characteristics of placebo medication but most is inconclusive. It seems that both very large tablets (because of their size) and very small tablets (because of presumed potency) are more effective than those of moderate size. The colour may be important according to the condition and a bitter taste is presumed more effective. Although pharmacologically inert, placebos may produce side-effects. These are usually mild e.g. drowsiness, nausea, and presumably based on previous learning and expectancy e.g. subjects told they are to receive alcohol and given placebo may report intoxication. However, the prescriber should be alert to more serious adverse reactions.

Clinician. A greater effect is shown when clinicians are authoritative, enthusiastic and really believe a particular treatment will work. This probably explains the large placebo effects found in clinical trials of new medicines and the success of unscientific, non-specific treatments.

Patient characteristics. All patients may show a placebo response under certain circumstances but no patient will consistently show a strong response. Research has shown that a placebo response is more likely in the young, those of lower intelligence or educational level, those with a desire to please, who cooperate with treatment or who are suggestible. Anxiety within the treatment situation is also important.

Condition. A placebo response is more likely in conditions where the symptoms are under cerebral control e.g. pain. Studies have indicated that whereas placebos can be very effective on the tolerance of pain, they do not affect the threshold. There is some evidence that subjects who responded to a placebo injection given to relieve dental pain, produced more endogenous opioid.

Both social and psychological aspects are therefore a very powerful part of any treatment. Doctors should not become preoccupied with outcomes expressed purely in biological or scientific terms to the exclusion of patient satisfaction and quality of life.

SUMMARY

The advent of the major psychotropic drugs in the 1950s led to major changes in the treatment of and attitudes towards people with psychiatric disorders. These have been largely beneficial but have also led to some over-prescribing for minor problems. Non-compliance with any treatment regime is a problem but is common with prescribed drugs. Compliance can be improved by education, behavioural intervention and strengthening the therapeutic alliance between doctor and patient. Any treatment can result in psychological dependence but stopping drug treatment may also involve withdrawal signs of physiological dependence. The placebo effect should not be underestimated in the treatment of psychiatric disorders.

FURTHER READING

Brewin, C.R. (1984) Perceived controllability of life-events and willingness to prescribe psychotropic medication. *British Journal of Social Psychology* 23, 285–287.

Brubacher, D. (1994) Aspects of compliance: a review. *Journal of Pharmaceutical Medicine* 4, 31–39.

Buchanan, A. (1992) A two-year prospective study of treatment compliance in patients with schizophrenia. *Psychological Medicine* 22, 787–797.

Busto, U. and Sellers, E.M. (1986) Pharmacokinetic determinants of drug abuse and dependence. A conceptual perspective. *Clinical Pharmacokinetics* 11, 144–153.

Chaput de Saintonge, D.M. and Herxheimer, A. (1994) Harnessing placebo effects in health care. *Lancet* 344, 995–998.

Conrad, P. (1985) The meaning of medications: another look at compliance. *Social Science and Medicine* **20**, 29–37.

Farré, M. and Camí, J. (1991) Pharmacokinetic considerations in abuse liability evaluation. *British Journal of Addiction* **86**, 1601–1606.

Gabe, J. and Bury, M. (1988) Tranquillisers as a social problem. *Sociological Reviews* **36**, 320–352.

Hallström, C. (ed.) (1993) *Benzodiazepine Dependence*. Oxford University Press, Oxford.

Mazzuca, S.A. (1982) Does patient education in chronic disease have therapeutic value? *Journal of Chronic Disease* **35**, 521–529.

Piatkowska, O. and Farnill, D. (1992) Medication — compliance or alliance? A client-centred approach to increasing adherence. In *Schizophrenia* (Kavanagh, D.J., ed.). Chapman and Hall, London.

Pringle, M. and Morton-Jones, A. (1994) Using unemployment rates to predict prescribing trends in England. *British Journal of General Practice* **44**, 53–56.

Rogers, A., Pilgrim, D. and Lacey, R. (1993) *Experiencing Psychiatry: Users' Views of Services*. Macmillan in association with MIND Publications, London.

Rollnick, S., Heather, N. and Bell, A. (1992) Negotiating behaviour change in medical settings: the development of brief motivational interviewing. *Journal of Mental Health* **1**, 25–37.

Scott, D.K. and Ferner, R.E. (1994) 'The strategy of desire' and rational prescribing. *British Journal of Clinical Pharmacology* **37**, 217–219.

Sellwood, W. and Tarrier, N. (1994) Demographic factors associated with extreme non compliance in schizophrenia. *Social Psychiatry and Psychiatric Epidemiology* **29**, 172–177.

Stainton Rogers, W. (1991) *Explaining Health and Illness: An Exploration of Diversity*. Harvester Wheatsheaf, London.

Webb, S. and Lloyd, M. (1994) Prescribing and referral in general practice: a study of patients' expectations and doctors' actions. *British Journal of General Practice* **44**, 165–169.

West, R. and Gossop, M. (eds) (1994) Comparing drugs of dependence. *Addiction* **89**.

Chapter 4

PHARMACOLOGICAL FACTORS IN DRUG TREATMENT

In this chapter we outline the complexities of the pharmacology of the drugs used in psychiatry. This touches on biochemistry, neurophysiology and neuroanatomy, as well as molecular biology. More detailed accounts are available in Leonard (1992) and Cooper, Bloom & Roth (1991). The subject can be divided into basic neuropharmacology, pharmacokinetics (the effects of the body on drugs) and pharmacodynamics (the effects of drugs on the body).

NEUROPHARMACOLOGY

In the last 50 years, the first neurotransmitters were discovered and mechanisms for their synthesis and breakdown were slowly identified. The pace of progress has since accelerated and the availability of highly specific radioactively labelled biochemicals has facilitated the identification of many different binding sites in the CNS, many of which have physiological functions (receptors).

The synapse is the junction between neurons and here electrical signals are transduced into chemical flows and back again. Drugs influence this junction through many mechanisms relating to neurotransmitters, including synthesis, release, breakdown and direct effect on receptors.

Synthesis, storage and release. The nucleus of the nerve cell contains deoxyribonucleic acid (DNA), which comprises the genetic information that controls the synthesis of all proteins, including enzyme molecules. The enzymes which synthesise the neurotransmitter are produced in the nerve cell body and are transported down the axon to the nerve terminal (Figure 4.1). The cell body and nerve terminals also take up into the neuron the appropriate precursor for synthesis of the particular neurotransmitter — choline, for example, in the case of those cholinergic nerves that release acetylcholine. The synthesised neurotransmitter is stored in thousands of specialised synaptic vesicles, or granules inside each nerve terminal (Figure 4.2).

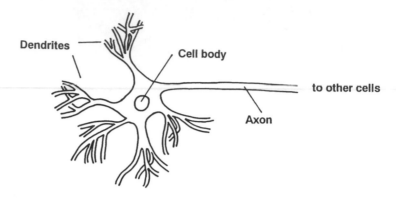

Figure 4.1   Schematic diagram of a neuron

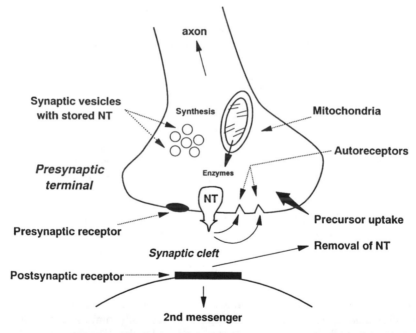

Figure 4.2   Diagram illustrating the main structures involved in the process of synaptic transmission. NT = neurotransmitter

After the nerve is activated, major flows of sodium and potassium occur across the membrane and propagate the nerve impulse. At the nerve terminal, calcium flow is involved and the storage vesicles then release their contents into the synaptic cleft.

Action on receptors. The synaptic cleft is narrow, so that the neurotransmitter rapidly diffuses across to the postsynaptic membranes, where it binds to specific protein receptors. Table 4.1 lists several classes of receptors. These are classified according to the main neurotransmitter, and further subtyped with specific chemicals ('ligands'). Binding of the transmitter to the receptor sets in train further biochemical events involving 'second messengers'. Ultimately a further electrical impulse is generated or, conversely, on-going activity is suppressed.

Inactivation and regulator mechanisms. If the transmitter were to activate the receptor permanently, neurotransmission would fail. Mechanisms must operate to remove the neurotransmitter from the receptors: the transmitter can diffuse away from the synaptic cleft with subsequent absorption into the circulation; active re-uptake may occur through specific uptake sites on the presynaptic membrane back into the neuron; enzymatic breakdown inactivates the neurotransmitter to inactive metabolites.

Important mechanisms regulate the synthesis of transmitters. Many neurotransmitter systems contain receptors on the presynaptic as well as on the postsynaptic membranes, and on the cell bodies themselves. Activation of these 'autoreceptors' inhibits further neurotransmitter release and synthesis. Thus, excessive traffic across the synapse diminishes the amount of neurotransmitter available which in turn lessens trans-synaptic activity. A second synaptic regulator mechanism involves the postsynaptic receptors. Underactivity across the synapse increases the numbers of receptors and their sensitivity. The converse also occurs: excessive trans-synaptic activity culminates in fewer available receptors ('down-regulation').

Sites of drug action. Several sites in and around the neuron are sensitive to drug effects.

1. Drugs can stimulate or block an enzyme in the synthetic chain.
2. Drugs can act as precursors, resulting in increased amounts of the natural neurotransmitter (e.g. L-tryptophan and serotonin).
3. The uptake and storage of neurotransmitters can be impeded resulting in depletion at the nerve endings (reserpine prevents dopamine storage).
4. The neurotransmitter can be released by a drug from storage granules (amphetamines release dopamine).
5. Drugs can block the enzyme in the neuron that destroys any free transmitter in the cytoplasmic fluid (MAOIs act here).
6. Conversely, some drugs act on the enzymes in the synaptic cleft, usually inhibiting them and thus prolonging the neurotransmitter's action.
7. The re-uptake of the transmitter into the presynaptic neuron can be blocked by some drugs (e.g. selective serotonin re-uptake inhibitors).

Table 4.1 Classes of receptor

Subtype	Location/function	Agonist	Antagonist
Cholinergic			
Muscarinic	Widespread CNS and	oxotremorine	atropine
Nicotinic	neuro-muscular junction	nicotine	α-bungarotoxin
Dopaminergic			
D_1	Stimulates adenylate cyclase	SKF 38393 analogue	antipsychotics
D_2	Inhibits adenylate cyclase	quinperole	sulpiride
Adrenergic			
Alpha$_1$	Postsynaptic	phenylephrine	prazosin
Alpha$_2$	Mainly presynaptic	clonidine	idazoxan
Beta$_1$	Cardiac stimulation	isoprenaline	metoprolol
Beta$_2$	Bronchodilation	salbutamol	IPS-339
Serotonergic			
5-HT$_1$	5-HT-labelled	buspirone	—
5-HT$_2$	Spiperone-labelled	—	ketanserin
5-HT$_3$	—	—	odansetron
GABAergic			
GABA$_A$	Affects chloride channels	muscimol (modulated by benzodiazepines)	bicuculline
GABA$_B$	?potassium channels	baclofen	
Opioid			
Mu	—	morphine	—
Delta	Receptor for enkephalins	—	—
Kappa	—	dynorphin	—
Sigma	—	phencyclidine	—

8. Many important drugs act directly on transmitter receptors either activating them directly (agonists) (e.g. benzodiazepines) or preventing the action of the natural neurotransmitter (antagonists) (e.g. beta-blockers).

No drug has a single isolated effect and most psychotropic drugs have a multitude of actions.

SPECIFIC NEUROTRANSMITTERS

Acetylcholine

Synthesis, storage and release. Acetylcholine is synthesised from choline and acetyl radicals by the enzyme choline acetyltransferase. Acetylcholine is stored in the synaptic vesicles. When an impulse arrives at the nerve ending, several hundred vesicles discharge simultaneously into the synaptic cleft. Calcium ions are essential for the process.

Inactivation. Body fluids and tissues contain cholinesterases that split acetylcholine into choline and acetic acid. Acetylcholinesterase is sited in neurons and hydrolyses acetylcholine rapidly.

Receptors. The receptors have been divided into the muscarinic (activated by the alkaloid muscarine) and the nicotinic (activated and later blocked by nicotine) types. Muscarinic activation results in a rapid action, whereas nicotinic activation is slower and more sustained. Both effects are produced by acetylcholine, but many drugs are fairly specific to one or the other type of receptor.

Pathways. Because techniques are limited, cholinergic pathways have generally been worked out using the identification of synthetic and breakdown enzymes and uptake and binding mechanisms for choline and acetylcholine. Cholinergic neurons occur widely in the brain and spinal cord and hence influence many neuronal and behavioural functions. One important pathway is that from the basal forebrain (e.g. nucleus basalis) to the cerebral cortex: these neurons degenerate in Alzheimer's Dementia.

Drug mechanisms. Many drugs block acetylcholinesterase, and increase and prolong the actions of acetylcholine. Physostigmine (eserine) is the prototypal cholinesterase inhibitor. Irreversible inactivators of cholinesterase were developed as insecticides and nerve-gas poisons and include the organophosphates such as parathion. Physostigmine has been used to treat Alzheimer's Dementia. Substances acting directly on cholinergic receptors include methacholine, carbachol, and the alkaloids, pilocarpine and muscarine. The most widely used cholinomimetic is nicotine from tobacco, but nicotine has complex actions. The antimuscarinic agents directly block acetylcholine (muscarinic) receptors and include alkaloids such as atropine and hyoscine, synthetic drugs such as propantheline, and the antiparkinsonian drugs such as benztropine and trihexyphenidyl. Some antipsychotic drugs such as chlorpromazine and thioridazine, and tricyclic antidepressants such as amitriptyline and prothiaden, also have powerful muscarinic-blocking properties.

Catecholamines

These include dopamine, an important neurotransmitter in the basal ganglia, limbic system, and other parts of the brain; noradrenaline (norepinephrine; NA), the transmitter in most sympathetic postganglionic fibres and certain tracts in the brain; and adrenaline (epinephrine), the major hormone of the adrenal medulla and also a central neurotransmitter.

Synthesis, storage and release. The precursor amino acid tyrosine is taken up into the nerve ending and hydroxylated to dihydroxyphenylalanine (dopa). This is converted to dopamine by the enzyme L-aromatic amino acid decarboxylase (sometimes called dopa decarboxylase). Dopamine enters the synaptic vesicles, which in noradrenergic neurons contain dopamine-beta-hydroxylase, which adds a hydroxyl group forming noradrenaline. Finally, in the adrenal medulla and in certain parts of the brain, noradrenaline is methylated to adrenaline.

The rate of synthesis of catecholamines depends on the amount of available tyrosine hydroxylase, i.e. this is the 'rate-limiting' enzyme. The catecholamines are stored in high concentration in the vesicles.

Inactivation. Dopamine and noradrenaline are removed from the synaptic cleft by re-uptake across the presynaptic membrane and thence into the storage vesicles. Enzymatic breakdown requires several enzymes, the most important being monoamine oxidase (MAO), widespread throughout the body, and catechol-o-methyltransferase (COMT). Dopamine is converted mainly to its acidic derivative 3-methoxy-4-hydroxyphenylacetic acid (also called homovanillic acid (HVA)). The metabolites of noradrenaline are more complex, the main ones being 3-methoxy-4-hydroxymandelic acid (vanillylmandelic acid, (VMA)) and 3-methoxy-4-hydroxyphenylglycol (MHPG).

Receptors. This topic is becoming increasingly complex. The two main types of dopamine receptors are the D_1 and D_2 families but D_3, D_4 and D_5 subtypes have been identified using molecular biology techniques.

The noradrenergic receptors are classified into alpha and beta categories. Alpha-adrenoceptors can be subclassified, alpha$_1$ adrenoceptors being postsynaptic and alpha$_2$ mainly presynaptic. The beta receptors in the periphery can be further divided into beta$_1$, chiefly at cardiac sites, and beta$_2$, which occur elsewhere, including the bronchi. Both alpha and beta adrenoceptors can be excitatory or inhibitory, depending on the location. The brain has both alpha- and beta-adrenoceptors.

Pathways. Dopamine receptors are found in the vomiting centre (area postrema): dopaminergic blockade exerts an important antiemetic effect. In the brain stem, dopaminergic neurons emanate from nuclei in the substantia nigra. The axons of these neurons form the nigrostriatal pathway, which innervates the caudate nucleus, putamen, globus pallidus, and, possibly the amygdala. This pathway degenerates in parkinsonism. Antipsychotic drugs produce the parkinsonian syndrome by competitively blocking the dopamine receptors on the cholinergic interneurons in the striatum.

The mesolimbic system terminates in the nucleus accumbens (just in front of the caudate), the olfactory tubercle, the septum, and related areas. This tract is believed to act in the regulation of emotional behaviour, especially its motor components. Other neurons project to the cerebral cortex, thus modulating higher cerebral function.

Another dopaminergic pathway inhibits the release of prolactin from the anterior pituitary. Thus, dopamine agonists lower prolactin concentrations in the body whereas dopamine antagonists such as antipsychotic drugs raise them.

Noradrenergic cell bodies are confined to the hindbrain, in the pons and medulla. The clearest cell-body grouping is the locus coeruleus, the 'blue site', situated in the floor of the fourth ventricle. It receives input from the periphery, and is responsible for noradrenergic innervation of all the cerebral cortices, thalamus, and all parts of the hypothalamus. Cells behind the locus coeruleus probably project to the cerebellum and yet another tract runs down into the spinal cord. Most noradrenaline release actually occurs away from synapses, fulfilling a 'neuro-modulatory' role, rather than being involved directly in neurotransmission.

Drug mechanisms. Drugs that interact with the synthetic enzyme tyrosine hydroxylase such as alpha-methyl-p-tyrosine impair the synthesis of dopamine and noradrenaline. Precursor administration increases catecholamine synthesis, provided that tyrosine hydroxylase is bypassed. Thus, administration of L-dopa increases the synthesis of dopamine in dopaminergic neurons and of noradrenaline in noradrenergic neurons. Concomitant administration of a dopa decarboxylase inhibitor such as carbidopa or benserazide which does not cross into the brain results in even higher brain concentrations of dopamine. This is the basis for the treatment of parkinsonism. The storage of catecholamines is disrupted by reserpine and tetrabenazine.

Many sympathomimetic agents act indirectly by displacing noradrenaline from its neuronal stores without impairing synthesis. Ephedrine, amphetamine and tyramine are important examples. The major inactivation pathway, re-uptake, is blocked by the tricyclic antidepressants and related drugs. These compounds affect catecholamines and serotonin (5-HT) re-uptake to varying extents: the re-uptake of dopamine is usually least impaired. Cocaine and amphetamine also inhibit re-uptake. Monoamine oxidase inhibition results in a failure to break down catecholamines which are then available for uptake into the stores and subsequent release. Monoamine oxidase exists in two forms, A and B.

Many drugs act directly on catecholamine receptors. Dopamine agonists include apomorphine, and bromocriptine, whereas the antipsychotic drugs are antagonists. Agonists on the alpha-adrenoceptor include noradrenaline and the directly acting sympathomimetic agents, phenylephrine and phenylpro-panolamine; beta-adrenoceptor agonists include isoprenaline and salbutamol. Phentolamine, some ergot alkaloids, and some antipsychotic agents such as chlorpromazine and haloperidol block adrenoceptors of the alpha type. Beta-adrenoceptor blockade is the main action of the large and important group of drugs such as propranolol.

5-Hydroxytryptamine (serotonin)

Synthesis, storage and release. The precursor of 5-HT is the amino acid tryptophan. Hydroxylation by the enzyme tryptophan hydroxylase to 5-hydroxytryptophan is the rate-limiting step. As concentrations of tryptophan are normally below optimal, the availability of tryptophan governs the amount of neurotransmitter synthesised. The 5-hydroxytryptophan is decarboxylated by L-aromatic amino acid decarboxylase to 5-HT.

Like the catecholamines, 5-HT is stored in vesicles at the presynaptic ending. Other tissues such as blood platelets can take up and store 5-HT.

Inactivation. Re-uptake into nerve terminals is the primary route of inactivation of 5-HT. The 5-HT can be broken down by monoamine oxidase, especially type A. The main metabolite is 5-hydroxyindoleacetic acid (5-HIAA).

Receptors. Multiple 5-HT subtypes have been characterised in the brain using a variety of techniques. New ones are described very frequently and cloning techniques from molecular biology have verified that they are distinct species of molecules. The best-defined are the 5-HT_{1A}, 5-HT_2 and 5-HT_3 subtypes.

Pathways. The serotonergic pathways stem from cell bodies situated mainly in the midline raphe nuclei. The upward projections provide diffuse innervation to the forebrain. Serotonergic fibres project from the raphe to the limbic system (hippocampus and amygdala), lateral geniculate, and superior colliculus. Another serotonergic pathway runs down from midline regions in the brain stem to innervate the spinal cord.

Drug mechanisms. L-tryptophan or 5-hydroxytryptophan administration increases 5-HT concentrations in the brain. Conversely, giving a drink containing all essential amino acids other than L-tryptophan results in 5-HT depletion. As with the catecholamines, reserpine depletes the nerve endings of 5-HT and prevents its storage.

The re-uptake of 5-HT into the presynaptic endings and vesicles can be blocked by some of the tricyclic antidepressants such as clomipramine and amitriptyline, but these drugs (or their metabolites) also block NA re-uptake. In the case of the selective serotonin re-uptake inhibitors, the re-uptake of 5-HT is selectively blocked without affecting NA. Monoamine oxidase inhibitors increase 5-HT concentrations by preventing the breakdown of the pool in the cytoplasm of the nerve.

Hallucinogens such as LSD and mescaline have complex actions on 5-HT systems. These drugs inhibit serotoninergic cell firing. Non-hallucinogenic analogues such as methysergide block both pre and postsynaptic receptors. Cyproheptadine is a potent 5-HT (and histaminic) receptor antagonist. Fenfluramine releases 5-HT from nerve endings. Recently, anxiolytics have been developed which act on 5-HT_{1A} receptors.

Gamma-aminobutyric Acid (GABA)

GABA was identified first as an important constituent of the crustacean nervous system and later of the mammalian central nervous system. GABA is a powerful inhibitor but progress has been slow because of the lack of drugs acting specifically on GABA mechanisms. It has been estimated that 40% of synapses in the brain are 'GABAergic', making GABA the most ubiquitous neurotransmitter.

Synthesis, storage and release. GABA is synthesised by decarboxylation of the amino acid glutamic acid by the enzyme glutamic acid decarboxylase (GAD).

The release of GABA in response to electrical stimulation is dependent on calcium ions.

Inactivation. Like the monoamine transmitters, GABA is taken back into the presynaptic nerve endings by a high-affinity uptake mechanism. Enzymic breakdown culminates in succinic acid which then re-enters the Krebs metabolic cycle.

Receptors. The brain contains many short interneurons, inhibitory in function with GABA being the usual neurotransmitter. GABA receptors have been classified as GABA$_A$ and GABA$_B$. The former are close to chloride channels across the nerve membrane so that GABA influences their opening. Benzodiazepines bind to this receptor at a site distinct from that of GABA. Thus, GABA stabilises the resting membrane potential producing inhibition, and benzodiazepines potentiate this effect.

Pathways. GABA nerve endings are involved in both presynaptic and postsynaptic inhibition in the spinal cord. These pathways seem in part to descend from the medulla and short interneurons also participate. The cerebellar cortex contains many GABA inhibitory neurons. Another GABA pathway originates in the caudate nucleus and terminates in the substantia nigra, exerting an inhibitory influence on the nigrostriatal dopaminergic neurons. GABA neurons are also widespread throughout the brain, including the cortices. Inhibitory influences are exerted on the noradrenergic locus coeruleus cells and the serotoninergic cells of the raphe nuclei. Dopaminergic (mesolimbic) and cholinergic projection pathways are also influenced by GABA inhibition.

Drug mechanisms. Some convulsants inhibit GABA synthesis, and many other drugs interfere with the GABA uptake mechanism. The anticonvulsant drug sodium valproate slows GABA breakdown by inhibiting succinic semi-aldehyde dehydrogenase. The alkaloid muscimol is a specific receptor agonist, whereas bicuculline and picrotoxin are receptor antagonists.

Other Neurotransmitters

The amino acid glycine is an inhibitory agent in the spinal cord. One of strychnine's actions is powerful antagonism of glycine receptors.

Glutamic acid and aspartic acid, both dicarboxylic amino acids, have widespread excitatory functions in the mammalian nervous systems and are now accepted as being neurotransmitters.

Some polypeptides have a neuroregulatory function. Some, such as oxytocin, vasopressin, luteinising-hormone-releasing hormone (LHRH), thyrotropin-releasing hormone (TRH), and growth-hormone-release-inhibiting hormone (somatostatin), are released by the hypothalamus and transported to the anterior pituitary, where they regulate endocrine secretions. However, these releasing factors are found in other neurons of the brain and may 'modulate' neurotransmission, i.e. modify neuronal responses to other neurotransmitters. Peptides found in the central nervous system include ACTH, substance P, neurotensin, vasoactive intestinal peptide (VIP), cholecystokinin, bradykinin, and angiotensin II. The central nervous system functions of these peptides, many of which were originally discovered in the gut, are currently being elucidated. Many are released in conjunction with the classical neurotransmitters such as NA. Specific binding sites for opioids have been found in the central nervous system, particularly in sites known to be associated with pain transmission. Specific narcotic antagonists such as naloxone also bind to these receptor sites with high affinity.

PHARMACOKINETICS

Pharmacokinetics comprises the effects of the body on drugs and relates to the way the drug reaches its site of action. Some knowledge of this topic is necessary in order to understand some important aspects of drug action. However, as much of pharmacokinetics is highly technical, this section is intended to outline some basic principles and to illustrate the relevance of these principles to psychotropic effects. Pharmacokinetic parameters provide essential information about the onset, duration of action and offset of single and repeated doses, the optimal dosage interval, the effects of physiological factors such as age and sex, and pathological disorders like liver and kidney failure, and the possibility of drug interactions.

The importance of inter-individual differences is emphasised in pharmacokinetics, both with respect to quantitative variability and qualitative idiosyncrasy. This is often relevant to treatment failures or to abnormal drug reactions.

Several drug parameters are usually cited. The *biological half-life* is the time taken for the biological effects of the drug to halve. As this decay in activity is usually exponential, this half-life is usually a constant, i.e. the time taken from full activity to half-activity is the same as that from half to quarter, and so on. The *plasma elimination half-life* is the time taken for the drug concentration in the blood to halve. It is constant for a given drug in a given individual, providing other metabolic factors such as alcohol intake, diet, etc. are unaltered. The half-life determines the dosage interval of a drug and the delay to achieving steady-state on repeated administration or complete elimination after stopping the drug. In both cases, the delay is four to five times the half-life.

The *apparent volume of distribution* (V_d) is a theoretical ratio reflecting the amount of drug in the body tissues as compared with plasma concentrations. For most psychotropic drugs the V_d is large because they are taken up avidly by bodily tissues such as the brain because they are soluble in fatty materials (high 'lipophilicity'). An exception is alcohol which is distributed evenly throughout the body.

The *total body clearance* is the fraction of the apparent volume of distribution which is cleared of the drug per unit time. It is an index of the rate at which the drug is eliminated from the body by whatever route.

The four processes which govern the pharmacokinetics of a drug are absorption, distribution, metabolism and excretion. They determine the three parameters outlined above but often in a complex way.

Absorption

Psychotropic drugs must penetrate to their site of action in the brain via the bloodstream, the main exception being the injection of drugs into the cerebro-spinal fluid. A drug enters the circulation either by being placed there by intravenous injection or by absorption from organs such as the gastro-intestinal tract, the lungs or the muscles (Figure 4.3).

The *intravenous* mode of administration results in a minimal delay before the drug can exercise its effects. It is easy to control especially if given by infusion rather than a rapid injection. The disadvantages are that transiently very high concentrations occur during injection, and once injected the drug cannot be easily removed.

Intramuscular injections are commonly used to facilitate administration. The rate of absorption depends on the blood flow through the muscles and this may be markedly increased during states of excitement. Long-acting *depot* injections comprise preparations of drugs like fluphenazine and flupenthixol which are highly fat-soluble as the decanoate or similar formulation in an oily medium. They are injected into muscular tissue from which they are slowly absorbed over the ensuing two to four weeks.

In the *oral* route absorption takes place from the gut. Absorption from the stomach and upper intestine is the most important but the location of the most rapid absorptive process depends on the chemical properties of the drug. Some drugs are absorbed rapidly from an empty stomach, alcohol for

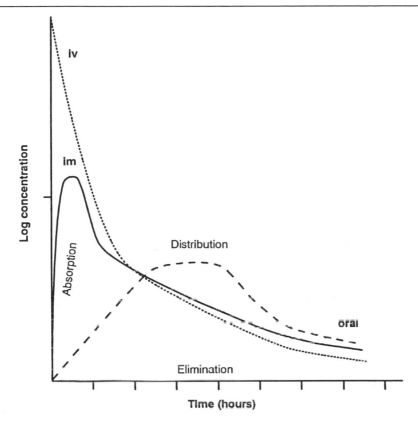

Figure 4.3   Schematic representation of the processes of distribution, absorption and elimination of a drug over time via the intravenous (IV), intramuscular (IM) and oral routes

example. However, a full stomach may impede absorption. Thus, for a rapid action a drug should be taken before meals, for a smoother, sustained action it should be taken after meals. Some drugs influence gastric emptying so can interfere with the absorption of other drugs given at the same time. Drugs can be formulated as sustained-release preparations: the drug slowly leaches out of an inert matrix.

Drugs can be given *sublingually* (under the tongue) and may be absorbed quite rapidly. The *rectum* is another place where absorption is efficient and suppositories are often used when the patient is vomiting.

Other routes of administration include inhalation, intra-nasal spray, ointments, lotions, patches etc. applied to the skin, eye drops, pessaries and ear drops.

Distribution

Drugs reach their target organs depending on the rate of blood flow through the organ and on the fatty solubility of the drug. Psychotropic drugs are generally highly fat-soluble, the brain has a rich blood supply, so entry to the sites of action should be quite rapid. However, the biological membrane between blood capillary and brain tissue is rather more complex than in other organs, giving rise to the 'blood-brain-barrier'. This is not, however, an absolute barrier and the rate of diffusion across it can still be rapid.

Another factor governing distribution in the blood stream is *protein binding*. Many drugs, including such psychotropic ones as the tricyclic anti-depressants, benzodiazepines and phenothiazines, bind to plasma proteins, mostly albumin, alpha$_1$-glycoprotein and globulins. This means that an appreciable proportion of the drug in the circulation is not in the plasma water but bound to the proteins in the blood, although in equilibrium with the 'free' drug. As binding can be high the effective concentration may be much less than the total concentration in the blood would suggest. Consequently, anything which alters the binding may have major implications; for example, one drug may displace another from its binding sites on the protein and thereby increase the effective plasma concentration.

Metabolism

Drugs which are relatively lipid-insoluble (e.g. barbitone) or highly ionised or elements (e.g. lithium) are excreted unchanged by the kidney. Most lipid-soluble drugs are readily reabsorbed back into the bloodstream from the glomerular filtrate in the kidney, i.e. their renal clearance is low. To be eliminated, drugs must be rendered less lipid-soluble, usually by metabolism mainly in the liver.

The main process is *oxidation*. Liver microsomal enzymes are usually involved although more specific enzyme processes may be important, for example, in the metabolism of alcohol to acetaldehyde and then acetic acid. *Conjugation* comprises the coupling of molecules such as sulphate and glucuronic acid to the drug to form less lipid-soluble complexes.

Psychotropic drugs, being lipid-soluble, undergo extensive metabolism with many metabolites, some of which retain psychotropic activity. Complex patterns occur which vary substantially among individuals.

Anatomical organisation dictates that drugs absorbed from the stomach and upper intestine must pass through the liver before entering the general circulation. The amount of metabolism as the drug passes through the liver after absorption from the gut is termed the 'first-pass effect'. It can be quite substantial with up to 90% of a drug being broken down before it can exert any effect (equals low 'bioavailability'). Intramuscular injections largely avoid this, which is part of the rationale for both standard and depot injections.

When more than one drug is administered, metabolic interactions can occur. Different drugs may compete for a common metabolic process leading to the *inhibition* of breakdown of one drug and its subsequent accumulation. A therapeutic example of this is the drug disulfiram which blocks the metabolism of acetaldehyde after the drinking of alcohol. The accumulation of acetaldehyde causes unpleasant symptoms which deter further drinking. Conversely, some drugs stimulate liver enzymes — *'drug induction'* — so that other drugs are metabolised more rapidly. Barbiturates are well-known inducers.

Liver diseases may affect drug metabolism, oxidation being more affected than conjugation. Drug metabolism becomes slower in the elderly, again particularly with respect to oxidative processes. Pregnancy also influences metabolism but distribution is also affected as the cardiovascular system alters markedly in function.

Excretion

Plasma water is constantly being filtered through the glomeruli in the liver, all but 1% being reabsorbed. Only free drug in plasma water can be filtered and only lipid-insoluble drugs and metabolites will fail to be reabsorbed. The acidity or alkalinity of the urine will influence excretion: amphetamine, a weak base, is excreted rapidly in acid urine; barbiturates, weak acids, are eliminated in alkaline urine.

Lithium is the main psychotropic drug excreted almost entirely via the kidneys. Thus, kidney failure can lead to accumulation of lithium with severe side effects culminating in death.

Drugs can also be excreted through the liver into the bile and then reabsorbed, the *enterohepatic* cycle. Other forms of excretion involve expired air, saliva, sweat and milk.

Pharmacological effects

The variability of drug response is well-known. The reasons for this variation relate to concentration and sensitivity. All the factors reviewed above govern the eventual concentration at the site of action, typically a population of receptors in the brain. However, the sensitivity of the tissue to the drug may also vary and the underlying factors are usually ill-understood.

Table 4.2   Some reasons for the monitoring of psychotropic drugs

Doubts about compliance
Therapeutic failure at usual dosages
Adverse drug reaction at usual dosages
Drugs with a narrow therapeutic range
Diagnosis of drug intoxications
Drugs likely to induce their own metabolism
Consequences of drug interactions
Consequences of diseases
Necessity to minimise plasma concentrations

Many attempts have been made to relate drug concentrations, usually in the plasma, to psychotropic and clinical response. Apart from lithium, these attempts have yielded rather disappointing results and routine monitoring of drug concentrations is uncommon. However, it may be helpful in certain situations (Table 4.2). Even where a relationship has been established across a group of subjects, the variability is still great and clinical decisions in individual cases not much helped. Adverse effects are often easier to correlate with plasma concentrations than are therapeutic responses.

PHARMACODYNAMICS

Factors Influencing Response

A wide range of factors influences the response of an individual to a drug (Table 4.3). Some of the more important are outlined below:

A. Dose

The effect of a drug varies with dose but sometimes in a complex way. The classic dose-response curve is S-shaped. There is no effect until a threshold dose is reached. Thereafter the effect increases with dose or with the logarithm of the dose until a plateau of maximal effect is attained. However, with some drugs such as the antidepressant, nortriptyline, further increases in doses are associated with a waning of effect which is therefore apparent over a restricted dose range, the 'therapeutic window'.

B. Multiple effects

No drug has a single action in therapeutic practice. Even at the subcellular level such as the synapse, drugs may interact with a number of processes

Table 4.3 Factors affecting drug response

Pharmacological	Dose
	Route of administration
	Duration of treatment
	Co-administration of other drugs
Individual	Age
	Weight
	Gender
	Pathology
	Diet

involving enzymes, uptake mechanisms and pre and postsynaptic receptors. Because many of the psychotropic drugs were discovered by accident, they tend to have multiple actions biochemically and therapeutically. For example, chlorpromazine is sedative, antipsychotic and antiemetic but can cause parkinsonism and other extrapyramidal reactions and can lower the convulsive threshold. Newer drugs designed to bind to only a few types of receptors tend to have fewer unwanted actions. Nevertheless, because a receptor type may be involved in neurotransmitter mechanisms governing a range of physiological functions, multiple effects may be inevitable. For example, the selective serotonin re-uptake inhibitors (SSRIs) are fairly specific to serotonin reuptake sites. Nevertheless, because serotonin is involved in so many functions, these drugs affect appetite, sleep, anxiety and compulsive phenomena as well as ameliorating depression.

C. Initial Level

The effect of a drug can be markedly influenced by the on-going activity of the system when it is given. This may cause 'paradoxical effects' in some subjects under some conditions.

D. Time Effects

These are also important. Single doses of a drug may give some indication of effects but the pattern and intensity of those effects may alter quite substantially on repeated administration. Tolerance to therapeutic and to unwanted effects is well-known, being a nuisance in the former instance but welcome in the latter. Examples include the lessening of sleep-inducing activity with regular use of sleeping tablets, and the lessening of sedation with some tricyclic antidepressants. After administration of drugs, abrupt discontinuation may be followed by rebound or withdrawal phenomena.

E. *Individual Variation*

Subjects vary considerably in their response to drugs and such variation can be seen right down to the subcellular level (Table 4.3). Factors such as gender, age, body type and nutrition profoundly influence drug response, as can the illness itself. Thus, studies in normal subjects can only give a rough indication of possible therapeutic effects although unwanted effects may be predicted more reliably.

F. *Milieu Effects*

Drugs are not usually given to individuals in isolation. The response of a patient may be different in hospital to in the community, e.g. larger doses of antipsychotics may be needed on an acute ward with several disturbed patients than in a quiet, supportive home atmosphere.

THE DEVELOPMENT OF NEW DRUGS

Clinical trials are now commonplace in most hospitals, both in-patients and out-patients being involved. As many psychotropic medications are mainly prescribed in primary care, general practice trials are also becoming common.

Although many factors enter into the efficacy and safety of medications, the development of new ones tends to follow well-tried but rather empirical paths. This reflects the accidental way in which many psychotropic drugs were discovered and the continuing difficulties relating clinical effects to biochemical and pharmacological profiles of activity. The first step is the synthesis of a new chemical entity (NCE) usually based on a known drug. The molecule is manipulated with three broad aims in mind: firstly, to endow it with the desired properties, e.g. both dopamine and serotonin blockade; secondly, to avoid properties which are unwanted and believed to underlie side effects, e.g. alpha$_1$ blockade and postural hypotension; thirdly, the drug should possess acceptable pharmacokinetic properties, i.e. not too short or too long an elimination half-life. It is of course essential that the drug can reach its site of action in the brain.

Next, the substance is tested in animal systems believed to predict clinical effects. Receptor binding studies are used to delineate the profile of receptor activities. Typically, strong binding is required to one or two types of receptor without binding to other putatively irrelevant receptors. For example, a drug developed as a 'pure' typical neuroleptic might be expected to bind to D$_2$ receptors alone. Animal models of drug action have long been a focus of controversy but they were potentially misleading — many of the early animal models for neuroleptic drugs detected possible extrapyramidal effects (movement disorders) rather than putative antipsychotic activity. Consequently, a whole generation of antipsychotic drugs inevitably caused extrapyramidal effects until it was realised that the two properties were separable.

The drug also undergoes toxicological screening in which it is administered to animals for both short and long periods to minimise the risk that it might have toxic properties.

The clinical development of a psychotropic drug is a complex and expensive affair. The animal models provide only a general guide to clinical efficacy although they are much more accurate in predicting side-effects. The usual groups of psychiatric patients investigated are probably heterogeneous, despite the care which has gone into developing modern diagnostic systems such as ICD-10 and DSM-IV. Placebo response is often quite high (30–50%), especially in the mildly ill patients, but it must be remembered that improvement combines both response to the administration of the dummy tablet and spontaneous improvement. Further limitations of sensitivity relate to the less-than-complete response to most psychotropic medications. The typical response rate of anxious, depressed or psychotic individuals to anxiolytics, antidepressants and antipsychotics respectively is about 60–80%. Thus, there is only a narrow 'window' between placebo and drug response in which to show drug–placebo differences should they exist.

The earliest phase of development (phase I) comprises the first administration of the drug to man. A very conservative dose is chosen, based on the effective doses in animal models. Escalating doses are given to a series of normal subjects until some effect is noticed. At the same time as seeking to detect clinical effects, simple pharmacokinetic readings are made, such as time of maximal blood concentration and elimination half-life. EEG studies may be informative at this juncture.

In phase II, a relatively small number of patients are exposed to the drug, often in flexible dosage. The type of patient is chosen from the profile of activity seen in animals. Efficacy is sought over an appropriate period, for example, six to eight weeks for an antidepressant, and placebo-controlled studies are routine now. Side-effects are carefully recorded. Unless good efficacy is found, the drug may be abandoned.

Phase III involves the greatest investment in time, money and number of patients. A set of coordinated clinical trials is designed to answer questions about the degree of efficacy, predictors of response, the range of indications, the frequency of the more common side-effects, dosage recommendations and so on. A series of smaller studies will address issues such as use in the elderly and perhaps children, those with liver or kidney failure, drug interactions, detailed psychological effects, etc.

When phase III is completed, sufficient information should be available to satisfy the appropriate governmental regulatory bodies. Further trials are usually promoted, so-called phase IV studies. These are primarily commercial in nature, for example, comparing the new drug with competitor products, looking at special tests, unusual groups of patients and so on.

The Role of the Regulatory Authorities

Until the 1960s, most countries did not regulate the introduction of new medications, the USA being the most notable exception. It was a therapeutic disaster involving a psychotropic drug, thalidomide, which resulted in first a voluntary and then a compulsory vetting procedure for new drugs. Statutory control has now burgeoned to the point that complaints are made that innovation is being stifled. In the UK in 1968, the Medicines Commission was appointed to advise on the supply and use of drugs. Under it, the Committee on Safety of Medicines was set up as an expert advisory committee to recommend the acceptance or rejection of new drug applications and to monitor side-effects. On completion of development for registration of a new drug, manufacturers are required to furnish detailed data on synthesis, chemistry, pharmacology, pharmacokinetics, toxicology, pharmaceutics, safety in human volunteers and clear evidence of efficacy. The side-effects and toxicology from a few thousand patients are also required as well as long-term tolerability data.

Efficacy is generally established using clearly-defined patient groups. The definition is based on acceptable criteria such as those of the ICD-10 or DSM-IV. Placebo-treated controls are usually incorporated in the study despite the proven efficacy of comparator substances in most psychotropic drug categories. This is because of the variability of response so that even well-established drugs may prove ineffective on occasion. This failure of efficacy is becoming a particular problem in trials run in primary care contexts using patients with milder illnesses.

The monitoring of adverse drug events is a difficult procedure because their nature is not easily predicted. Minor adverse reactions are common with 40% or more of patients reporting some side-effects with most types of medication. In the somewhat artificial conditions of a controlled clinical trial, the reporting of an adverse event can be closely scrutinised and further investigations instituted as appropriate. It is much more difficult to evaluate an apparent side-effect reported under normal clinical practice. Data are often incomplete or even fragmentary and the yellow card system of notification to the CSM markedly underestimates true incidences. The classical way of establishing causation is to re-challenge the patient with the drug, preferably with double-blind placebo control challenges as well.

Post-marketing surveillance is being used increasingly to establish the rare adverse event profile of a drug. A system of monitoring is set up to collate adverse reactions, usually reported to the general practitioner with the extent of use of the drug, as indicated by prescription data. This is usually instituted on initial marketing of a new drug.

More recently, with the advent of more expensive medications such as clozapine, attempts have been made to set drug treatment into a wider economic setting. Cost–benefit analyses have been carried out but their conclusions have often been disputed usually because of some of the cost assumptions made and also because some factors are difficult to cost. Attempts to persuade the prescriber to be more critical include regular patient reviews, audits, and notification of the time costs of a particular treatment or procedure.

The ethical aspects of drug development have also come under scrutiny as part of the wider debate on animal and human experimentation. Drug trials in patients have to be approved by a properly constituted and conducted Ethics Committee, usually within the institution, university or hospital, under whose auspices the study will be run. The issue of properly informed consent is particularly thorny with psychotropic drugs given to psychotic or demented individuals whose capacity to give adequately-informed consent may be doubtful. The consent of relatives is often needed but practice varies from country to country.

The Controlled Clinical Trial

The core element of a drug development programme, and indeed more widely the assessment of any treatment, is the controlled clinical trial. This has several essential elements:

1. The inclusion of carefully selected patients usually on the basis of a definable disorder but occasionally on a syndromic or even symptomatic basis. Minimal criteria of severity have to be met.
2. The rigorous exclusion of patients not meeting these criteria.
3. The random allocation of each individual patient to one of the available treatments. This is done on a 'blind' basis so that the investigator cannot influence which patient gets what.
4. The matching of active treatment to control or dummy treatment and to a comparator treatment if included. This is relatively easy in drug trials but more difficult in assessments of non-drug treatments where it is readily apparent that one treatment involves different elements than another. At the least, the treatments should be equated for therapist experience and

time. Even with drug treatments, complications can arise, e.g. comparing oral with injectable medication. Then, the 'double-dummy' procedure is resorted to: one group of patients is given active oral medication and a placebo injection, the other group receives oral placebo and active injection.

5. Adequate, relevant and reliable assessments are made at appropriate intervals. In trials of psychotropic drugs, relatively few objective measures are available or, if extant, are poorly validated. Rating scales are routinely used, of which there are many, e.g. Hamilton Anxiety and Depression Scales.

6. The assessments are made under double-blind conditions, i.e. neither the investigator nor the patient is aware of which treatment has been given. This may be difficult to ensure in practice because the characteristic side-effects of the drug may unblind the assessor. For example, in a comparative trial of an SSRI antidepressant and a tricyclic antidepressant, it is a fair guess that patients complaining of nausea are more likely to be taking the SSRI, those with dry mouth the TCA.

7. Finally, the data are analysed using appropriate statistics. Although this is the final stage, it is essential that statistical advice is sought at the outset. This will comprise checking the design of the study. In particular, the statistician can advise on the numbers of patients in each group which is needed to establish the drug–placebo difference with fair confidence, if it indeed exists: this is the so-called 'power' of the study. At the end of the study, the statistician will evaluate and analyse the data and establish whether the drug and control have effects which differ significantly, i.e. beyond the chance level, usually of 1 in 20 (0.05; 5%).

SUMMARY

Neuropharmacology is both a complex and rapidly expanding field of study. We have tried to give a brief outline of the factors involved such as synaptic transmission and the main neurotransmitters. The pharmacology of drugs can be divided into pharmacokinetics, the effects of the body on the drug, and pharmacodynamics, the effects of the drugs on the body. Pharmacokinetics comprises absorption, distribution, metabolism and excretion and explains how the drug gets to its site of action. Pharmacodynamic properties can be studied at several levels such as the biochemical and clinical but relationships between the two are often tenuous. The development of new drugs is strictly regulated and relies ultimately on controlled clinical trials.

FURTHER READING

Andreasen, N.C. (1988) Brain imaging: applications in psychiatry. *Science* **239**, 1381–1388.

Bloom, F.E. (1990) Neurohumoral transmission and the central nervous system. In *The Pharmacological Basis of Therapeutics*, (8th edn) (Gilman, A.G., Goodman, L. and Gilman, A., eds). Pergamon Press, New York, pp. 244–268.

Cooper, J.R., Bloom, F.E. and Roth, R.H. (1991) *The Biochemical Basis of Neuropharmacology*. Oxford University Press, New York.

Fuller, R.W. (1992) Basic advances in serotonin pharmacology. *Journal of Clinical Psychiatry* **53**:10 (suppl.), 36–45.

Harrington, M.A., Zhong, P., Garlow, S.J. et al. (1992) Molecular biology of serotonin receptors. *Journal of Clinical Psychiatry* **53**:10 (suppl.), 8–27.

Humphrey, P.P.A., Hartig, P. and Hoyer, D. (1993) A proposed new nomenclature for 5-HT receptors. *TiPS* **14**, 233–236.

Leonard, B.E. (1992) *Fundamentals of Psychopharmacology*. Wiley, Chichester.

Nedergaard, O.A. (1988) Catecholamines: regulation, release and inactivation. *Pharmacology and Toxicology* **63** (suppl. 1), 5–8.

Nicoll, R.A. (1988) The coupling of neurotransmitters to ion channels in the brain. *Science* **241**, 545–553.

Schimerlik, M.L. (1989) Structure and regulation of muscarinic receptors. *Annual Review of Physiology* **51**, 217.

Sieghart, W. (1992) GABA$_A$ receptors: ligand gated Cl ion channels modulated by multiple drug-binding sites. *TiPS* **13**, 446–450.

Spoont, M.R. (1992) Modulatory role of serotonin in neural information processing: implications for human psychopathology. *Psychological Bulletin* **112**, 330 350.

Strange, P.G. (1991) Interesting times for dopamine receptors. *Trends in Neuroscience* **14**, 43–45.

Tuominen, M. and Leppaluoto, J. (1987) Peptides and neurotransmission in the central nervous system. *Medical Biology* **65**, 137–142.

Willner, P. (ed.) (1991) *Behavioural Models in Psychopharmacology*. Cambridge University Press, Cambridge.

Zetler, G. (1985) Neuropharmacological profile of cholecystokinin-like peptides. *Annals of the New York Academy of Science* **448**, 448–469.

Chapter 5

PSYCHOLOGICAL MEASURES USED TO ASSESS DRUG EFFECTS

In this chapter we describe ways in which drug effects can be recorded. Because psychotropic drugs exert their main effects on the brain, it is important to determine not only desired mood changes but also potential performance or memory impairment. The sort of rating scales and tasks which are used are described.

It is not sufficient to compare psychotropic drugs on clinical efficacy alone. To administer a drug is to introduce an independent variable which may affect numerous different aspects of an individual's functioning. A full evaluation with a number of measures examining these potential effects is therefore necessary. A drug may be safe and effective therapeutically with few obvious side-effects to the clinician, but it may still exert subtle dysphoric effects or impair skills that are necessary for adequate functioning in a complex technological society. Psychological methods may be used to detect these undesirable effects as well as those that may be desirable and thus by alerting both doctor and patient, reduce the potential harmful consequences. There are two main ways of gathering information: subjective, i.e. what the subject tells us and objective, i.e. the subject's performance on various tasks.

METHODS OF RECORDING SUBJECTIVE DRUG EFFECTS

Recording subjective effects of psychotropic drugs is very important because these drugs are usually administered to alter how the patient feels. Although this chapter is primarily looking at how to measure subjective effects induced by a drug, this is inextricably linked to how the patient, or indeed subject, feels before drug administration. Early drug studies followed the psychology of the time and used introspection, i.e. the experimenter administered the drug to him/herself and recorded its effects. This method is still occasionally used by experimenters to evaluate substances with unknown or unpredictable effects. A classic example is that of Albert Hoffman and LSD. This then

Table 5.1   Methods of recording subjective drug effects

Adjective checklists
Semantic differential
Visual analogue scales
Rating scales
Questionnaires

developed into administering the drug to other people and asking them how they felt before and after consumption. The problem with such open-ended approaches is two-fold. Firstly what is the meaning of the subject's response, e.g. 'I feel woolly', and secondly how does it compare to another subject's 'I feel spaced out'. To combat this, more standardised methods of measuring subjective effects have been developed (Table 5.1). However, it is important to recognise that greater standardisation limits the amount of information that a subject can give. Adjective checklists started as lists of adjectives, e.g. good, happy, tense, irritable, sleepy, which the subject was asked to endorse if they applied to him/her. The semantic differential is a technique which has been used to put opposing adjectives at either end of a scale, e.g. good–bad. The subject then rates him/herself on a seven-point scale between the two adjectives. Visual analogue scales abolish the seven points and allow subjects to rate anywhere between the two adjectives on a 10 cm line, thus effectively allowing 100 points. These scales have been shown to allow frequent estimation of feelings or side-effects, are sensitive to change, practical and reliable. Some versions of multiple scales have been subjected to factor analysis to allow groupings of scales measuring the same factor, e.g. sedation.

Numerous rating scales and questionnaires have also been developed to measure mood states, e.g. depression, or personality. These are not intended to measure drug effects *per se*, rather therapeutic changes brought about by the drug. Therefore measures of clinical efficacy usually relate to a particular mood state or disorder. They aim to measure the severity of a clinical state which has either been diagnosed according to a classification system or which has been identified as a problem. This state is expected to respond to a specific intervention, e.g. a drug. Some of the commonly used scales are set out in Table 5.2. The items within a scale will differ according to the theory underlying its construction. Thus although both the Hamilton Depression Rating Scale (HDRS) and the Beck Depression Inventory (BDI) purport to measure depression, the HDRS is based on the biological theory of depression, whereas the BDI is based on the cognitive theory. Thus the HDRS is more likely to be used in studies evaluating drugs and the BDI in studies evaluating cognitive therapy, and this can be a problem when comparing different treatments. In studies setting out to evaluate the

Table 5.2   Some examples of observer rating measures of clinical efficacy

Scale	Condition
Positive and Negative Syndrome Scale	Schizophrenia
Scale for the Assessment of Positive Symptoms	Schizophrenia
Scale for the Assessment of Negative Symptoms	Schizophrenia
Hamilton Depression Rating Scale	Depression
Montgomery–Asberg Depression Rating Scale	Depression
Beck Depression Inventory	Depression
Hamilton Anxiety Rating Scale	Anxiety
Clinical Anxiety Scale	Anxiety

combination, both scales should be used as although the total scores have been shown to correlate quite highly ($r = 0.7$), there may be differential responsiveness across items.

METHODS OF RECORDING OBJECTIVE DRUG EFFECTS

There are two main purposes in recording the objective effects of psychotropic drugs. The first aim is to determine the types of function they may impair or improve and how people consuming these drugs will be affected in their daily life. The second aim is to use the drugs to tell us more about psychiatric or psychological phenomena, to improve theoretical models of memory, for example. However for the purposes of this book, the discussion will be confined to the first aim as this has direct relevance to mental health care. Psychotropic drugs may affect alertness, attention, concentration, motor performance and cognitive processes as well as feelings. To study these effects various types of performance task are used. These can broadly be discussed under four headings: perceptual, psychomotor, attention and cognitive processes.

Assessment of Perceptual Functioning

Perception is the process we use to try and interpret all the information which comes to us from our various sense organs. Although perception refers to all senses, by far the greatest amount of work has been done on vision. It is possible to study both the threshold and the speed of perception. One of the most often used techniques in drug studies is the *critical flicker fusion threshold*. This can be defined as 'an intermittent light subjectively perceived as a steady light if the frequency of flashes is increased above a certain limit'. It is usually measured by the method of limits with fusion and discrimination rates determined during a number of increases and decreases of frequency. It has been found to be sensitive to both sedative and stimulant drug effects. Another method of assessing perceptual processing is *tachistoscopic display*. This measures the speed or extent of processing rather than the threshold but has fallen into disuse because early experiments did not find significant effects. Similarly, *after-image* has not proved sensitive. In contrast to these, the measurement of eye movements via electro-oculography has increased in use since the development of microprocessor-based systems. Both *smooth pursuit* and *saccadic eye tracking* are particularly sensitive to psychotropic drug effects but saccadic eye movements are also able to show onset, duration and tolerance effects.

Assessment of Psychomotor Performance

A large number of methods are available for recording motor performance. These were developed to study the effects of various variables on human performance in occupational psychology and thus provide a readily available resource for studying drug effects. Factor analytic studies have, however, failed to find a factor of either general psychomotor skill, manual dexterity or physical proficiency but have identified a number of unitary abilities which can all be measured by various tasks. Psychomotor performance may be assessed by pencil and paper tests and by apparatus. These methods range from a simple reaction time task to a complex work sample test, e.g. operating machinery. It is not possible to discuss all the different types of task here but some examples are given in Table 5.3. It is important to recognise that most of the tests involve more than one psychomotor ability component. The recording of body sway or ataxia with microprocessor-controlled instruments has been recommended as requiring very little subject cooperation.

Assessment of Attention

Attention is a key feature in psychological testing as if information is not attended to, it can neither be responded to, nor remembered, nor learned. It is

Table 5.3   Examples of psychomotor tasks

Finger tapping
Reaction time
Pegboard
Trail making
Body sway
Balance beam

thus involved in all tests but certain tests have been devised to measure it directly. These range from simple short scanning tasks, e.g. *cancellation* of a particular number in a series of numbers to similar but longer tasks using a fixed rate of display of numbers or letters on a computer screen when the subject has to press a key in response to a particular stimulus as in the *continuous performance task*. These rapid information processing tasks can be made more complex by varying the number or pattern of stimuli requiring a response. Tests that require sustained attention over a long period of time in order to detect irregularly occurring rare events are called *vigilance* tasks. Such tasks are particularly applicable to some jobs, e.g. operators of complex, automated systems, but because of their length of administration, cannot form part of a test battery.

Assessment of Cognitive Processing

The term cognitive here refers to the higher functions of learning and memory. Memory is central to human cognitive abilities and the measurement of drug-induced changes in memory perhaps represents the area of most growth and sophistication. Memory can be understood to encompass three components: sensory, short-term and long-term. Sensory memory refers to very brief sensory impressions for each modality. Short-term memory is also known as primary or working memory. It only stores information for very brief periods of time. Active rehearsal or consolidation is required to transfer information to long-term or secondary memory. The processes of learning and memory can be broken down into three main stages:

1. *acquisition* which involves information intake (registration) and processing (encoding),
2. *storage* which involves retaining the information in memory,
3. *retrieval* which is necessary to reproduce the information.

Retrieval can be tested by either recall or recognition. A drug may be given prior to acquisition or prior to retrieval to test effects on these processes. Although theoretically it could be given between acquisition and storage, in reality this process may only take seconds and thus is much faster than the action of any currently available psychotropic drugs. A drug which disrupts acquisition processes is said to produce *anterograde amnesia*, i.e. reduced learning of new information following treatment. A drug which disrupts retrieval may produce *retrograde amnesia*, i.e. loss of information learned prior to treatment. Secondary memory can also be divided into *declarative* (explicit) and *nondeclarative* (implicit). Declarative memory represents records of experiences which can be explicitly retrieved. Nondeclarative represents knowledge of skills (procedural) or priming responses. Declarative memory can be further subdivided into episodic and semantic. Episodic memory consists of memories for personal experiences and contains a context whereas semantic memory is generic and contains knowledge of facts and language. There are various memory tests to measure different facets of memory processing. Some examples are given in Table 5.4. Although psychiatric disorders may impair different components of memory, psychotropic drugs seem to show most impairment on episodic memory.

Neurophysiological Measures

The effects of psychotropic drugs on higher CNS functions can also be evaluated by neurophysiological methods. Electroencephalography is an important diagnostic tool in neurology. It can therefore measure the effectiveness of anti-convulsant drugs on epileptic seizures. It is not a very precise measure of drug effects in psychiatric disorders but certain drug groups can be shown to exhibit characteristic EEG profiles. Because the EEG wave pattern changes from the waking to sleep state, several sleep stages can be differentiated (Chapter 8) and the effects of drugs on these described. Waveforms related to stimuli such as brief tones and flashes of light and to responses such as a key-press can also be used to assess the effects of some drugs. These waveforms are called 'evoked responses' or 'event-related potentials'.

The advent of brain imaging techniques in humans has already yielded interesting results and technical advances should provide important data about brain function and drug action. Positron emission tomography (PET) involves the administration of esoteric radio-active substances manufactured in a cyclotron. These substances are 'ligands', that is, they bind to specific

Table 5.4 Examples of memory tasks related to memory processes

Memory Process	Task
PRIMARY	Digit span
SECONDARY Nondeclarative (Implicit)	Skill learning Priming
Declarative (Explicit) Episodic	Personal memory Word recall
Semantic	Category generation

receptor sites in the brain. The localisation and degree of occupancy of those receptors can then be visualised using special sensitive radiation detectors and complex computer analyses. For example, it has been shown that during antipsychotic drug therapy, 70–85% of dopamine receptors have to be occupied for a clinical effect. Single photon emission tomography (SPET or SPECT) is similar but simpler technically. Magnetic resonance imaging (MRI) does not use radioactive substances but relies on intrinsic properties of the spin of some atoms, usually hydrogen. All these techniques can be adapted to yield measures of regional blood flow in the brain.

EVALUATION OF EFFECTS

Normal Subjects Versus Patients

Nearly all studies investigating the effects of psychotropic drugs on performance use healthy volunteers. This means subjects who are physically and psychiatrically healthy at the time of testing and who are not taking any medicines. Usually an interview is also conducted to try and establish that the subject has never suffered from any significant physical or psychiatric disturbance. The subject's GP may also be contacted. Many studies are conducted in university settings, meaning the healthy subjects are often students, a highly selected group, even less representative of the general population. Many studies early in drug development only use male subjects because of the possibility in women of an unplanned pregnancy with potential risk to the foetus. This limits their applicability even further. There are now moves to include women so that important potential gender differences in the clinical pharmacological profile of a drug can be studied. Likewise more studies are examining drug effects in specific groups, e.g. the elderly, because they are known to be more sensitive to adverse events. However the major problem is not the sex nor age of the subject but the generalisability of results in healthy volunteers to a psychiatric patient population.

Studies in healthy volunteers are valuable for several reasons. They allow precise, controlled measurement of performance changes pre- and post-drug. This enables us to determine which functions are potentially improved or impaired by a drug rather than the illness or therapeutic response. They also give an indication of the duration of action of a single dose and they allow detection of significant side-effects. However, in general, healthy volunteers experience side-effects and performance decrements at much lower doses than those which are clinically prescribed and frequently results indicating impairment in healthy volunteers have not been replicated in patients. This is partly due to the fact that psychiatric patients often exhibit impairment on a range of psychological tests due to their condition and consequently a therapeutic response to a drug, e.g. decreased anxiety, may result in task improvement rather than impairment. This scenario is even more likely with repeated doses. Therefore although studies in healthy volunteers may help in the planning of therapeutic trials, they are no substitute for studies in the clinical population for whom the drug will be prescribed.

Acute Versus Repeated Doses

As well as using healthy volunteers, most drug studies use only a single acute dose of a drug. While again this may give us an indication of what to look for, it bears little relationship to the clinical situation in which two to three doses may be given a day for periods of weeks or months. Multiple doses can at least show us a dose response curve but repeated dose studies are needed to see if tolerance develops to any performance impairment while maintaining the therapeutic response. In general any impairments decrease with repeated administration even in healthy volunteers but it is necessary to be alert to the possibility of cumulative effects or the persistence of effects after drug termination.

Test Selection and Sensitivity

In order to obtain precise and objective evidence of a drug's effects, it is necessary to use a battery of psychometric tests, sampling a variety of functions. The tests used should be sensitive to both improvement and impairment of functioning. They should be appropriate to the clinical population who will be prescribed the drug and face validity tends to improve motivation. Each individual test in the battery should be brief to avoid excessive fatigue and parallel forms should be feasible to allow repeated testing in order to evaluate change. At one time it was assumed that complex processes would show more effect than simple tasks. However, complex technical systems do not necessarily show more effect and simple repetitive tasks often reveal impairment produced by sedative drugs. Intelligence tests like the Wechsler Adult Intelligence Scale (WAIS) have fallen into disuse because of their lack of discriminatory power although some subtests from the scale are frequently used, e.g. *digit symbol substitution test; digit span*. Tests of well-established functions or old learning, e.g. computational tasks, tend to show less impairment than those involving new learning, e.g. paired associates. Some reviewers have tried to produce a compilation of the most sensitive tests but these are usually confined to the effects of one group of drugs and such conclusions can be distorted by both the tendency to try and replicate significant findings and to publish only significant results. Batteries which combine tests of sedation, attention and memory can carry out analyses to separate out these effects although this has only rarely been attempted. It is important to point out the sensitivity of simple subjective measures such as visual analogue scales to both stimulating and sedating drug effects. These often detect effects at lower doses and show more consistency than objective measures. This may be because they are less affected by non-specific factors such as previous experience, practice and motivation.

Automated Testing

The rapid growth in information technology and microcomputers has led to the automation of various tests. Significant correlations between the standard test and the automated version have generally been found. However there is a tendency for scores on some automated versions to be lower, meaning it is not appropriate to use the standard norms nor to switch from one version to another. Computerisation minimises experimenter bias and time by standardising presentation and incorporating scoring. It also enables a more detailed task analysis to be performed on-line.

Non-specific Factors

Non-specific factors such as previous experience are often neglected in drug studies. Yet medical students' previous need to memorise large amounts of information may mean not only that they perform better on rote learning tasks, altering the ceiling level, but that they are also able to compensate for sedative drug effects on such tasks. In a similar way, subjects who regularly consume relatively large amounts of alcohol are likely to be less affected by benzodiazepines. A subject's motivation may also be influenced by repeated testing or boring tasks and this may be seen as an improvement in performance on the last testing of the day. On the other hand, some drugs may actually affect a subject's motivation to perform tasks efficiently. It may be very difficult to control such factors but it is important to be aware of their contribution to the overall pattern of results.

Interaction with Other Substances

Most drug studies rule out any concomitant medication but may not be as meticulous with common substances such as caffeine and nicotine or even food consumption. Many studies have looked at the combination of alcohol with various psychotropic drugs. In general, older drugs showed additive effects but many newer compounds do not interact. The psychotropic effects of nicotine and caffeine are well researched but despite this, few studies have examined the effects of these substances in combination with drugs. Many studies decide to exclude the consumption of caffeine-containing beverages on the study day but this may lead to increased tiredness and the confusion of withdrawal effects of caffeine with acute effects of the drug. In the same way asking subjects to starve for several hours may be necessary to obtain a fast onset of action and a good pharmacokinetic profile, but its effects on feelings and performance should not be overlooked.

The problems of drug interactions can be seen clearly in hospital accident and emergency units and clinicians should always be aware that acute states of confusion or delirium may have been caused by excessive or multiple drug use, whether intentional or accidental. The elderly are particularly at risk because not only are they more likely to have problems with their physical health which are then treated with other drugs, but they are also more likely to suffer from brain disease, and increasing age is associated with alterations in drug metabolism and disposition. However, it also occurs in those abusing other substances, e.g. alcohol, or those using over-the-counter (OTC) medicines. The latter problem is likely to become more prevalent as more prescription drugs become available OTC and people are encouraged to self-medicate for minor complaints.

Relevance of Laboratory Research

The relevance of acute dose studies in healthy volunteers to repeated use in psychiatric patients has already been discussed. However the relevance of the actual tests used has also been questioned. Many laboratory tests are stated to be analogues of real-world behaviours, e.g. driving, but their correlation with real-world tasks has rarely been investigated. Batteries of laboratory tasks often require maximal effort in speed and accuracy which is rare outside the laboratory. In real-life people tend to pace themselves and organise their work to compensate for any perceived inefficiency. One example is memory. Memory tests that have been used in drug studies have been criticised as being unrepresentative of everyday memory requirements. Everyday remembering does not usually involve deliberate attempts to store information. People remember personally relevant facts or things that are meaningful to them. Therefore lists of unrelated words are unlikely to be easily remembered. Studies which have looked at memory for more meaningful information, e.g. being taken to the operating theatre after an intravenous injection of a benzodiazepine or presenting words as a shopping list have generally found that drug-induced impairment was reduced.

To try and make other tasks more relevant, simulators have been used or studies have been conducted in applied situations. Several large scale trials were conducted by military organisations during the Second World War which generally showed that stimulants (caffeine and amphetamines) improved performance in real-life military duties. Recently, military research has concentrated on recreational substance use and its potential for impairment. Alcohol was deemed to cause the biggest problem. Car driving represents the applied area in which the greatest amount of drug research has been done. Various closed-course driving tests have been used during which variables such as manoeuvring, cornering, speed and care can be assessed. Open-road, dual-control driving has also been used in the Netherlands during which driving was assessed by advanced driving certificated examiners using a 110-item checklist. In general, those drugs which impaired driving under these conditions have also demonstrated impairment on laboratory performance tasks, and those not found to impair driving have not been found to impair laboratory tests, providing some validity for the latter.

Another approach to the study of drug-induced impairment in real-life involves epidemiological investigations of accidents. These may imply drug intake from self-report, prescription monitoring or drug levels in body fluids. These studies have implicated alcohol and psychotropic drugs with a sedative action as being associated with an increased likelihood of accident especially in the elderly in whom multiple drug use is more common. However, one review cautioned that although CNS stimulants generally improve performance they may also have a role in causing accidents. It is important to recognise that these studies suffer from many uncontrolled variables and that those studies which have attempted most control and have used a reference group, e.g. who were driving at similar locations and times to those at which accidents occurred, have not consistently demonstrated that psychotropic drugs increase accident risk in road traffic accidents. There is a need for more well-controlled epidemiological investigations both in the workplace and on the road.

In real-life situations, individuals determine their own interaction with the environment. If they perceive a drug-induced impairment, they may compensate for it by slowing down, avoiding certain activities like driving and using external aids like written reminders. The drugs that are likely to cause most risk to the user and others are those that impair judgement of abilities.

SUMMARY

All psychotropic drugs affect both mood and performance. It is important to determine if the benefits of a drug outweigh the risks. Any drug-induced changes must be measured reliably and accurately so that treatments can be compared. Observer rating scales and questionnaires have been developed to determine therapeutic changes brought about by drug treatments. Many different tasks are available to evaluate drug effects on psychological processes. Nearly all studies investigating psychotropic drug effects on performance are conducted in healthy volunteers. Although these studies are valuable, they are no substitute for studies in the appropriate clinical population.

FURTHER READING

Ellinwood, E.H. Jr. and Nikaido, A.M. (1987) Perceptual-neuromotor pharmaco-dynamics of psychotropic drugs. In *Psychopharmacology: The Third Generation of Progress* (Meltzer, H.Y., ed.). Raven Press, New York, pp. 1457–1466.

Hindmarch, I. (1980) Psychomotor function and psychoactive drugs. *British Journal of Clinical Pharmacology* **10**, 189–209.

Hindmarch, I. and Stonier, P.D. (eds) (1987) *Human Psychopharmacology. Measures and Methods* vol. 1. John Wiley, Chichester.

Hindmarch, I. and Stonier, P.D. (eds) (1989) *Human Psychopharmacology. Measures and Methods* vol. 2. John Wiley, Chichester.

O'Hanlon, J.F. and de Gier, J.J. (eds) (1986) *Drugs and Driving*. Taylor & Francis, London.

Squire, L.R. and Butters, N. (1992) *Neuropsychology of Memory* (2nd edn). Guilford, New York.

Spiegel, R. (1989) *Psychopharmacology. An Introduction*. John Wiley, Chichester.

Tulving, E. (1983) *Elements of Episodic Memory*. Oxford University Press, New York.

Chapter 6

THE COMBINATION OF DRUG AND PSYCHOLOGICAL TREATMENTS

Clinically, drug and psychological treatments are not administered in isolation. They are often combined but there is little research from which to predict the effects. The purpose of this chapter is to review the principles underlying the evaluation of combination therapies. The theoretically possible advantages and disadvantages of combining treatments are described. Methods of investigating these possible effects as well as methodological problems which may be encountered are outlined. The risk/benefit ratios of the component therapies are compared and the discussion is confined to treatments given simultaneously.

DRUG TREATMENT

The treatment of psychiatric disorders remains a clinical art based on an empirical and inexact science. Most research activity in drug treatment is focused on elucidating the parameters of treatment in terms of dose, duration of treatment, precise indications and so on (see Chapter 4). Factors such as double-blind conditions and matched placebo controls are considered essential, and it is accepted that the randomised controlled trial is the most powerful research design to assess the effects of a treatment. In response to this, drug companies have now introduced their own strict monitoring procedures in addition to those of the regulatory authorities. Even so, there is little control over less specific factors such as clinician and milieu. Patients participating in clinical trials usually see the same clinician on each visit and are allocated more time and attention than in standard practice which may explain the often considerable placebo effects. Results of treatment trials carried out in hospital out-patient settings as opposed to GP settings may produce more favourable results because extraneous variables are more easily controlled. In reality, the response of a patient to a particular drug depends on a variety of factors including side-effects, previous drug and illness history, and age. Clinical management, a non-specific, uncontrolled type of psychotherapy, sometimes described as 'supportive', always accompanies the administration of a drug. Drugs cannot be administered in isolation.

PSYCHOLOGICAL TREATMENT

Psychological treatments are varied in the specificity of techniques and in therapist orientation. Therefore the treatment which a patient receives may depend on the therapist they are referred to rather than their condition. Although there may be some agreement among professionals or in the literature about which treatment would be suitable for which disorder, this is not borne out in practice. Treatment is dependent on the referrer, the patient and the availability. Because of the large number of different types, research into non-pharmacological therapies is inchoate. Few studies have been carried out with adequate rigour concerning controls and blindedness. Many studies have used symptomatic volunteers and not clinically representative populations. The most common control groups have been no-treatment or waiting-list and where attempts at placebo treatments have been made, different therapists and contact time have often been used. Although behavioural forms of psychotherapy such as exposure and, more recently, cognitive therapy, have been evaluated in a more systematic way, the use of concomitant medication is rarely excluded or even controlled. In one recent comparison of cognitive therapy, analytic psychotherapy and anxiety management training in the treatment of generalised anxiety disorder, 68% of the patients were initially taking some form of psychotropic medication: 37% anxiolytics or hypnotics, 25% antidepressants and 6% both, but no attempt was made to look at the possible interactions with therapy. This was despite the fact that a reanalysis of an earlier similar study suggested that concurrent benzodiazepine treatment might interfere more with behaviour therapy than cognitive therapy. Nevertheless, several meta-analyses have shown that behavioural and cognitive therapies are more effective than psychoanalytic or humanistic therapies. The latter were generally found to be superior to minimal or no treatment conditions. The emphasis is now on isolating the important factors within each treatment so that the most effective treatment package may be constructed. For example, in the treatment of agoraphobia it has been found that exposure produces the most rapid change in avoidance but paradoxical intention reduces the frequency of panic attacks.

When different psychological treatments are compared within the same study, the situation is often difficult to interpret. In evaluating a psychological therapy, for example, the alternative intervention is often not used to full effect. This may be due to ignorance or unfamiliarity with the alternative treatment or to theoretical bias but it undoubtedly accounts for the disparate results in comparisons of cognitive therapy and behaviour therapy, for example.

Comparison of Drug and Psychological Treatments

When treatments not only from different theoretical bases but also from different disciplines are compared, bias is much more likely. A number of studies have compared the relative efficacies of drug and psychological treatments but explorations of the comparison and interactions between drug and non-drug treatments are rife with methodological weaknesses (Table 6.1). It is apparent in the literature that comparative and combination studies executed at centres favouring either drug or psychological therapy invariably find results in favour of their preferred treatment. This has been attributed to inadequate dose levels or lack of maintenance drug therapy on one hand and a lack of adequate training or therapist matching on the other hand. Such fundamental flaws can be illustrated by studies in depression. One of the first major trials to compare the tricyclic antidepressant, imipramine, to cognitive therapy in the treatment of depression was conducted at the centre at which cognitive therapy was developed. Understandably cognitive therapy was found to show greater change and less attrition than imipramine after 12 weeks' treatment. However, this study was flawed in several respects. Assessments were not conducted blind to treatment condition, imipramine doses were marginal and medication was tapered towards discontinuation two weeks prior to the final assessments. Thus the depression scores of patients on imipramine actually rose over the final two weeks of the study, contributing to the significant differences found between treatments at the end.

Such flaws are not confined to research on depression. Likewise, a study comparing psychological therapy with a benzodiazepine in the treatment of generalised anxiety systematically reduced the drug dosage through the trial. The study compared cognitive behavioural therapy, anxiety management training and lorazepam with a waiting list control. The authors state that although lorazepam produced most immediate and greatest improvement, these effects reduced as the trial progressed. However, these results would be

Table 6.1   Common methodological weaknesses

Inadequate dose levels or titration
Inadequate therapist expertise
Different therapist contact time
Non-blind assessments
Uncontrolled symptom severity

predicted from the design of the trial. Although patients assigned to both psychological therapies received two treatment sessions a week over four weeks, those assigned to lorazepam were prescribed a scheduled reduction in dosage (Figure 6.1). The study was thus testing gradual withdrawal after an acute 10 day phase of treatment.

Both these studies were examples of inadequate drug treatment. However, the reverse criticism has also been made of other studies. A major study comparing cognitive behavioural therapy, interpersonal therapy and imipramine with placebo found imipramine to be the most and cognitive therapy the least effective of the active treatments. A subsequent analysis showed this to be true only for those who were severely depressed and that these results were confined to one of the three participating sites. This has led to a questioning of the expertise and supervision of the therapists conducting cognitive therapy at that site. One reviewer has commented that outcome studies should aim to administer all treatments with equal enthusiasm and that psychological interventions must be provided by competent therapists. The same rule applies to drug treatment. A study comparing patients drawn from both GP and out-patient clinic settings found cognitive therapy to be superior to treatment with tricyclic antidepressants only in the GP setting. This has been attributed to a possible inadequate management of drug therapy by the GPs. It is impossible to judge this as no mean doses or dosage ranges were reported but it does highlight the importance of expertise in pharmacological as well as psychological treatment. Studies must be sound in their planning, execution and interpretation. To that end, it would seem important to have experts from both disciplines to advise on these facets of combination treatment trials. It is not sufficient for researchers and clinicians to increasingly

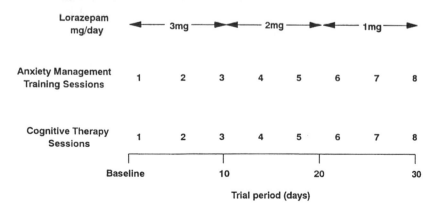

Figure 6.1 Treatment schedules in a study comparing psychological and drug treatment in generalised anxiety

rely on the statistical power of meta-analysis. Such techniques cannot correct faults in the clinical trials on which they are based and they often fail to exclude studies which are basically flawed, thus reducing the power of fundamentally good studies.

THERAPEUTIC APPROACHES

Six main ideological and philosophical approaches can be identified within psychiatry as described in Chapter 2. They comprise:

1. the disease or biological,
2. the psychodynamic,
3. the social or interpersonal,
4 the behavioural,
5. the cognitive,
6. the humanistic.

These models are identified with certain types of treatment (Table 6.2). Perhaps the latter might also encompass many of the alternative therapies favoured by lay people and practitioners but with little theoretical basis, e.g. acupuncture, hypnotherapy.

There are few psychiatric disorders which fit clearly into any one model as discussed in Chapter 2. Only the aetiology of the organic psychoses is distinctly biological. However this model has dominated the approach to

Table 6.2   The relationship of theory to treatment

Model of psychiatric disorder	Treatment examples
Biological	Drugs Electroconvulsive therapy
Psychodynamic	Analytic psychotherapy
Social/interpersonal	Interpersonal therapy Family therapy Group therapy Marital therapy
Behavioural	Graded exposure Systematic desensitisation Applied relaxation
Cognitive	Cognitive therapy
Humanistic	Client-centred therapy

other psychotic disorders. Because of their profoundly disturbed behaviour such patients were often incarcerated in institutions before the advent of the antipsychotic drugs. The effectiveness of these drugs reinforced the biological model, although the aim of caring for such patients in the community has led to extensive research into the contribution of social and psychological factors, and a more integrated approach.

In anxiety disorders, an equivalent impact has been made by both pharmacological and behavioural treatments. There are clearly advantages and disadvantages to both approaches. Medication is readily available, easy to deliver and acts relatively quickly. It also has side-effects and works only during administration or until natural remission takes place. Psychological therapy requires a trained practitioner, commitment to treatment and practice by the patient and takes longer to work. Its effects do not stop on termination and there are no side-effects. However, as these therapies are mainly given by people with different theoretical biases and training (Table 6.2), professional relationships have become involved, in some countries to the point of demarcation disputes. Objectively, we have evidence from many sources that both biological and psychological factors interact in the cause and treatment of a wide variety of physical illnesses and it is therefore important to tailor the treatment to the patient. In psychiatric or psychological disorders, this is much more important. No technique will help all patients and we need to know which patients respond best to which treatment and whether some patients require a combination of treatments.

TREATMENT COMBINATIONS

The theoretically possible advantages and disadvantages of the combination of treatments has been described in the literature. Three outcomes are possible on combining treatments: positive effects, negative effects and no effects (Table 6.3). Each is based on several different scenarios.

A. Possible Positive Effects

1. Drugs may make compliance with psychological treatments more likely. Patients seek treatment to relieve their distress. They are more likely to comply with a quick-acting treatment, which demands little time and effort. Many patients present for treatment at a time when they feel their self-efficacy is diminished. The rapid symptomatic improvement with anti-anxiety compounds, or on a longer time-scale with buspirone may reinstitute the patient's confidence in his/her coping strategies so that he/she perseveres

Table 6.3 Theoretical advantages and disadvantages of the combination of treatments

A. Positive effects

    1. Drugs increase psychological compliance
    2. Psychological treatments increase drug compliance
    3. Treatments act synergistically on different aspects

B. Negative effects

    1. Drugs can reduce symptoms so patient loses motivation
    2. Drugs may interfere with psychological treatments
    3. Drugs may distort therapist-client relationship
    4. Giving drugs is a complex act needing psychological exploration
    5. Stopping drugs is a complex act needing psychological help

with psychological treatments, behavioural, cognitive or dynamic. Likewise the improvement of motivation and concentration with antidepressant drugs may enable the patient to complete tasks or examine the links between past experiences, current thoughts and feelings.

2. Psychological treatments may improve drug compliance. Support, encouragement and explanation can facilitate the imbuing of confidence in the patient concerning the efficacy of the medication prescribed. Behaviour therapy includes education about specific techniques. Charting improvement in activities and symptoms may encourage the patient to persevere with drug treatment.

3. Various treatments may act synergistically on different aspects of the disorder. For example, in a patient with panic attacks and agoraphobia, drug treatments can suppress the panics, behavioural treatments can modify the behaviour. In schizophrenia, an antipsychotic drug may improve hallucinations and delusions while social skills training and family education aid rehabilitation into society.

B. Possible Negative Effects

1. Drugs can reduce symptoms to the point where the patient loses motivation to persist with psychological treatments. Benzodiazepines may produce an immediate anxiolytic and a mild euphoric effect resulting in symptomatic comfort and reluctance to pursue other treatments. Antidepressants may relieve depression to the extent that the patient does not wish to remember the previous feelings and has no desire to try and

recognise the link with negative thoughts.

2. Drugs may interfere with psychological treatments because of impairment of learning, memory and concentration. Drugs might then impair the effectiveness of behaviour therapy. In the most extreme form, state-dependent learning may occur. New learning would not generalise from the drug state to the non-drug state so psychological improvement would be lost when the drug was discontinued.

3. Drugs may distort the therapist–client relationship. A drug may have a negative placebo effect by increasing dependency on the therapist. The patient assumes a passive role in therapy and feels no need to persist with the planned psychological therapy. The expectation is that the doctor will cure them and they take no responsibility for their own role in the disorder.

4. Giving drugs is a complex act needing psychological exploration. If drug effects are the focus of any patient/therapist interaction, the therapeutic process may develop into a search for the right medication irrespective of other factors such as relationships or life events. The patient may feel their self-efficacy is further reduced and fail to persist with any psychological goals. Any improvement will be attributed to the medication regardless of other factors.

5. Stopping medication may present problems. It is important to taper both anxiolytic and antidepressant medication. Concern has been expressed over the dependence potential of long-term drug use, in particular with benzodiazepines, and discontinuation may need the mobilization of intensive non-drug therapies. Psychological dependence may ensue after any drug which has produced symptomatic improvement, even placebo.

C. No Interactions

This is the null hypothesis that carefully designed studies are set up to refute. One assumes that the two (or more) therapies simply add up in their effects without interacting (Table 6.4). If they do interact, they may potentiate, i.e. the effects of both together is greater than the sum of the parts, or alternate, either one or the other being effective, or subtract, one treatment interfering with the other as above. A modification to the 'alternate' interaction may apply if one of the treatments is known to be more effective than the other. The effect of the two combined may equal the individual effect of the more potent and this has been called 'reciprocity'.

In effect, two fully adequate treatments combined may produce little or no greater benefit than each treatment alone. This may be because of a ceiling effect: such treatments already mobilise the patients' recovery potential to the full. However, in this case, it is important to examine both the instruments used to measure improvement and the long-term outcome. For example, the combination of an antidepressant and cognitive therapy may produce no

Table 6.4   Combination treatments

	Type of interaction
1. Potentiate	$X + Y \rightarrow f(X + Y)$
2. Neutral	$X + Y \rightarrow X + Y$
3. Alternate	$X + Y \rightarrow X$ or Y
4. Subtract	$X + Y \rightarrow -f(X + Y)$

greater effect on clinician ratings of symptoms but may produce more improvement in self-efficacy or life-style. Likewise, there may be no difference between the combination and the individual treatments alone at the end of therapy but the improvement may be maintained for longer after treatment termination or may even prevent relapse.

Practical Considerations

Some practical considerations are important. Because drug and non-drug treatments may be administered by different people, liaison between them is important to avoid misunderstandings. Any hostility between them will be quickly sensed by the recipient who will lose first confidence and then patience with an invidious situation. If the patient sees a psychologist for behavioural or cognitive treatment and a physician for drug treatment, the ideal situation is for the patient, psychologist and physician to work as a therapeutic triad. All participants in this triad must communicate openly to avoid misunderstandings or therapeutic conflict. In practice, patients are often referred for psychological therapy with no mention of concomitant drug treatment. Likewise they may attend their GP during the course of a trial of psychological therapy and be prescribed a new drug or have the dose of a current drug altered. Psychological treatment trials often fail to ask about possible concomitant medication, whether this is prescribed or self-administered. In a survey of therapy, it was reported that psychologists treating agoraphobic patients with behaviour therapy were often unaware that they were taking two or more drugs at the same time. Obviously, a change of drug dosage or time of administration may affect factors in psychological therapy just as psychological techniques such as uncovering deep-seated problems, improving critical relationships or setting goals may affect response to a drug.

A second issue concerns the attitudes of the patient to various forms of therapy. Many patients are quite sophisticated in their knowledge of the types of treatment available and have marked preferences. Foisting a treatment on them to which they have objections, practical or theoretical, may result in the prompt default of the patient. As this therapeutic area has unfortunately tended to become polarized, some patients are unwilling to accept one or other component, thereby biasing the results of systematic studies.

METHODS OF INVESTIGATION

The nub of the investigation is to find out if and how the component treatments interact in combined therapy. To that end it is necessary to compare the combination with each of the factors of the combination delivered separately, i.e. with the appropriate control as well as with the combination of the controls (Figure 6.2). This approach involves a factorial 2×2 design in which each patient receives two 'treatments', one pharmacological and one non-pharmacological. However, each treatment is either active or placebo. This design is quite powerful as long as the placebos are well chosen. To make the design more powerful, it would be necessary to add two more groups: active drug alone and active psychological treatment alone. However, a six-cell design requires 50% more patients, which is probably not feasible in availability of suitable patients, time or costs.

Methodological Considerations

Even if a study is designed well according to the four-cell plan, certain methodological requirements must be met (Table 6.5). The main problem in conducting such a study is devising a placebo psychological treatment. Some researchers setting out to do this in comparative rather than combination studies have found that 'placebo' psychological treatments such as self-help

Drug

		Active	Placebo
Psychological treatment	Active	Both active	Psychological
	Control	Drug	Both inactive

Figure 6.2   Design of study investigating treatment interaction

packages or non-directive counselling are as effective as more structured approaches like cognitive therapy. Simple supportive measures similar to GP contact are a possibility but, in order to balance the design, these must be equivalent in number of sessions and contact time to the active psychological treatment package, in the way that a drug placebo must match the active treatment in every way except the content of the active drug. Many studies have merely evaluated drug plus psychological treatment versus drug plus standard care or management but this does not tell us whether it was the specific therapy which interacted with the drug or merely the additional time and attention devoted to the patient. It is also important that the same therapist administers both active and control treatments. However, even where this is controlled, one therapist may differ in his/her efficacy at administering a particular treatment. Attempts have been made to control therapist expertise by the use of treatment manuals. In reality one therapist may be more effective at administering any therapy, drug or psychological, because of other more humanistic factors, e.g. rapport, empathy, warmth.

Another important consideration is the selection of subjects. It is important that they are matched on initial severity and that they are not prescreened and rejected as being unsuitable for behaviour therapy or non-responsive to drug treatment on the basis of past treatment.

Previous treatment should be recorded. Patients who have had previous courses of psychological treatment may respond more quickly to a 'refresher' course. It is also important to specify how long patients must be free of any previous medication. If patients are taken off a benzodiazepine and included in a study using another drug, this may be either beneficial or detrimental depending on cross-tolerance.

When conducting a combination trial, the length of treatment is very important. Many drug trials of anxiety or depression last only four to six weeks but this may not be long enough to assess the effectiveness of a psychological therapy. Outcome measures should include those relevant to

Table 6.5   Important methodological considerations

Placebo controls
Therapist expertise
Subject selection
Previous treatment
Length of treatment
Outcome measures
Independent assessor
Times of evaluation

both drug and psychological therapies as often results on different outcome measures favour different treatment modalities, e.g. self-esteem improving with cognitive therapy, relationships with interpersonal therapy, and sleep and appetite with drug treatment.

In addition the assessor should be independent and not the person administering treatment. It has been shown that the person giving either drug or psychological therapy is biased to seeing improvement with it and will rate more favourably than an independent person blind to treatment with no investment in the outcome.

The time of evaluation is especially important in combination studies. Many studies have only evaluated the acute phase of treatment and have found drug and psychological treatments to be equivalent in the short-term with a swifter onset of action for the drug. The combination produces similar or marginally better results. However, another important question in clinical practice is 'does the patient remain well?' Short-term treatment generally has little long-term effect but psychiatric disorders may persist. The majority of patients with depression have recurrences and many anxiety disorders are chronic. It is therefore important to evaluate combination therapy over longer time-periods, to do regular follow-up assessments and possibly to evaluate additional refresher sessions of psychological therapy after drug discontinuation as there is evidence that this prolongs remission in depression. A future aim should be to see if new episodes can be prevented.

In conclusion, the number of studies addressing the issue of the efficacy, safety and clinical indications for combining pharmacological and psychological treatments is lamentably small. But this should not surprise us in view of the difficulties in conducting such studies in a rigorous way. Unfortunately most of the studies which have been completed suffer from methodological weaknesses, and very few have fulfilled the stringent criteria outlined here. This has led reviewers in the field to emphasise the necessity of further carefully designed studies. On the whole there are some indications that combined treatments are more effective than either alone but such differences are neither large nor robust. Additional studies with larger sample sizes could give definitive answers, in particular whether they may lead to a greater chance of complete recovery. More research effort should be expended in defining the parameters of such combinations. More educational effort should be expended in teaching the use of such therapies and more of our clinical effort should be spent in using such combined therapies in an integrated way. However, it is important that patients are also given an integrated treatment rationale.

SUMMARY

The randomised, controlled trial is the most powerful research design to assess the effects of a treatment. Most drug studies now conform to these standards. Research into psychological treatments is much less controlled. Many studies use waiting-list or no treatment controls. Comparative and combination studies suffer from many methodological weaknesses. Theoretically there are three possible outcomes from combining treatments: positive, negative and no effects. An investigation should be designed to find out if and how the component treatments interact in combined therapy by using a factorial 2 × 2 design, in which each patient receives two treatments, one drug and one psychological.

FURTHER READING

Beitman, B.D. and Klerman, G.L. (eds) (1991) *Integrating Pharmacotherapy and Psychotherapy*. American Psychiatric Press, London, U.K.

Durham, R.C., Murphy, T., Allan, T., Richard, K, Treliving, L.R. and Fenton, F.W. (1994) Cognitive therapy, analytic psychotherapy and anxiety management training for generalised anxiety disorder. *British Journal of Psychiatry* 165, 315–323.

Gray, J.A. (1987) Interactions between drugs and behavior therapy. In *Theoretical Foundations of Behavior Therapy* (Eysenck, H.J. and Martin, I., eds). Plenum, New York.

Hollon, S.D., Shelton, R.C. and Davis, D.D. (1993) Cognitive therapy for depression: conceptual issues and clinical efficacy. *Journal of Consulting and Clinical Psychology* 61, 270–275.

Hollon, S.D., Shelton, R.C. and Loosen, P.T. (1991) Cognitive therapy and pharmacotherapy for depression. *Journal of Consulting and Clinical Psychology* 59, 88–99.

Kahn, D. (1990) The dichotomy of drugs and psychotherapy. *Psychiatric Clinics of North America* 13, 197–208.

Kendall, P.C. and Lipman, A.J. (1991) Psychological and pharmacological therapy: methods and modes for comparative outcome research. *Journal of Consulting and Clinical Psychology* 59, 78–87.

Klerman, G.L. (1984) Ideological conflicts in combined treatment. In *Ideological Conflicts in Combined Treatment* (Beitman, B.D. and Klerman, G.L., eds). Spectrum, New York.

Klerman, G.L. (1986) Drugs and psychotherapy. In *Handbook of Psychotherapy and Behavior Change* (Garfield, S.L. and Bergin, A.E., eds). Wiley, New York.

Michelson, L.K. and Marchione, K. (1991) Behavioral, cognitive, and pharmacological treatments of panic disorder with agoraphobia: critique and synthesis. *Journal of Consulting and Clinical Psychology* 59, 100–114.

Tyrer, P., Seivewright, N., Murphy, S. et al. (1988) The Nottingham study of neurotic disorder: comparison of drug and psychological treatments. *Lancet* ii, 235–240.

Wardle, J. (1990) Behaviour therapy and benzodiazepines: allies or antagonists? *British Journal of Psychiatry* 156, 163–168.

Chapter 7

TREATMENT OF ANXIETY

In this chapter, the treatment of anxiety disorders is discussed. Benzo-diazepines comprise the major group of anti-anxiety drugs and their mode of action, clinical uses and drawbacks are outlined. Alternative drug treatments include buspirone, beta-blockers and antidepressants. Structured psychological approaches to anxiety are described as well as the effects of combining drug and psychological therapy.

Anxiety is a common human emotion, which is experienced in response to danger or threat and can best be conceived as a dimension ranging from normal to pathological. It is a feature of most psychiatric disorders but the major classification systems divide pathological anxiety into a number of separate disorders. These disorders have in common both psychological features, e.g. apprehension, worry, fear, and physiological manifestations, e.g. sweating, increased heart rate, trembling (Figure 7.1). They are differentiated by when these symptoms occur (Figure 7.2). In generalised anxiety disorder (GAD) they are present all the time although the degree and pattern may show considerable fluctuation and the disorder tends to be chronic. In phobic states, anxiety is evoked by certain, well-defined situations or objects. Simple phobias may be life-long but may not cause significant distress if the situation is rarely encountered. More complex phobias like agoraphobia or social phobia, however, may result in chronic avoidance and social isolation. In post-traumatic stress disorder (PTSD), the response to an exceptionally stressful or life-threatening event is delayed or protracted. In addition to the subjective and physiological symptoms of anxiety, the event is persistently re-experienced in images, thoughts and flashbacks. Panic attacks are discrete periods of intense fear or discomfort accompanied by numerous somatic symptoms. If these attacks are associated with specific situations, this may lead to avoidance or agoraphobia. If the attacks are recurrent but not associated with particular events, then a diagnosis of panic disorder (PD) may be made. Because significant anxiety occurs, obsessive compulsive disorder (OCD) is classified as an anxiety disorder. However, the key features are obsessional thoughts or compulsive acts. Obsessional thoughts are recognised as the patient's own thoughts but are both intrusive and

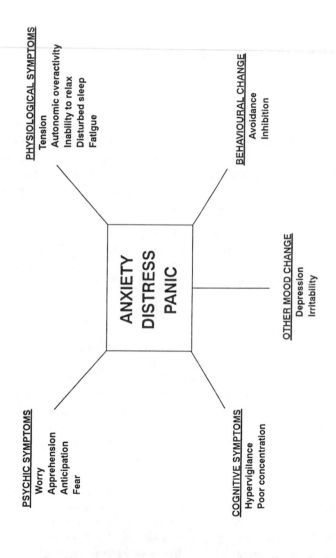

Figure 7.1 Features of anxiety

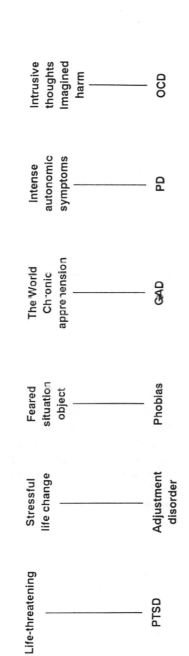

Figure 7.2 Precipitants of anxiety disorders

distressing. Compulsive acts or rituals are stereotyped, repetitive behaviour performed in order to prevent perceived harm. If resisted, anxiety is increased. Cormorbidity among the anxiety disorders and with depression is common.

SEDATIVES AND ANTI-ANXIETY DRUGS

The term 'sedative' originally meant a substance which had the ability to allay anxiety, i.e. have a calming effect. However, the meaning has shifted to imply feelings of drowsiness or torpor, a state which was originally called 'over-sedation'. The older compounds kept their rubric as sedatives, whereas newer drugs, meprobamate and the benzodiazepines, were dubbed 'tranquillisers' or 'anxiolytics' with the implication that they assuaged anxiety without inducing drowsiness. As will be seen, no such clear distinction can be made, except perhaps with the very newest anti-anxiety compounds, which act in a different way from their predecessors. We will use the term 'anti-anxiety drug' in preference to other terms, as this emphasises the purpose for which these medicines are prescribed without prejudging their actual profile of activity.

The Barbiturates

Although obsolescent in many respects, the barbiturates are still widely used as hypnotics, sedatives and anti-epileptic compounds, especially in Third World countries where they provide a cheap alternative to the benzodiazepines. They were first discovered at the turn of the century, barbitone, a long-acting compound, being the first, followed by phenobarbitone and at least 50 others. Barbiturates vary in their ability to cross biological membranes and hence enter the brain. Methohexitone sodium (Brietal) was used at one time to induce a state of relaxation: it was given by intravenous injection and had a very rapid effect. It is short-acting so the effects wear off in an hour or two. At the other extreme is phenobarbitone, used both as a sedative and an anticonvulsant. This drug is quite slow to penetrate the brain but it is also long-acting. In between are a range of medium-acting compounds used as sedatives. Amylobarbitone (and the sodium salt, amylobarbitone sodium) is the best-known. It will tend to accumulate to some extent as its half-life is around 15–20 hours. Barbiturates cross the placental barrier into the fetus and are also excreted in breast milk.

The barbiturates reversibly depress the activity of all excitable tissues. In the brain, barbiturates bind to specific receptor sites on the $GABA_A$ ionophere, potentiating the effects of GABA in inhibiting neuronal activity. However, in high concentration, barbiturates are believed to affect neuronal activity directly, not via GABA inhibitory mechanisms. This may explain why the barbiturates are toxic in overdose, producing excessive depression of neuronal activity in the respiratory and cardiovascular centres.

The effects of barbiturates range from mild sedation to general anaesthesia, depending on the dose. Some have anticonvulsant properties and many are powerful hypnotics. They lessen anxiety but at the cost of sedation. They depress respiration even in normal doses, particularly in individuals who already have breathing problems. They interact with many other drugs because they stimulate enzymes in the liver which metabolise these drugs (the P_{450} cytochrome system). Hence the actions of other drugs may be reduced or vitiated.

Many adverse effects involve neurological and psychological function and are strongly dose-related. Psychomotor impairment is noticeable and at high doses, slurred speech and impairment of eye movements are common. Dizziness, unsteadiness, weakness of muscle tone, double and blurred vision are all frequent complaints and complications. Unwanted psychological effects comprise drowsiness, heaviness, euphoria, restlessness and irritability. In some individuals, paradoxical excitement may ensue. In the elderly, confusion and memory disturbance are hazards. On chronic use, cumulation can occur with slowing down, decreased attention span, difficulty in thinking, poor memory, impaired judgement and even paranoid ideas. Some patients become disinhibited and emotionally labile.

Dependence is quite common and is usually manifest by steady increase in dosage and in a physical withdrawal syndrome when attempts are made to discontinue. As the dose is pushed up, signs of barbiturate intoxication occur with slurred speech, staggering gait and somnolence. On withdrawal, anxiety, insomnia, muscle weakness and trembling are routinely seen, together with anorexia, loss of weight and general physical debility. Fits, delirium and even death can occur, particularly when high doses are abruptly discontinued. Sometimes chronic hallucinations follow withdrawal in long-term users. Passive dependence can supervene in utero in the fetus of a mother taking barbiturates in late pregnancy. Most cases of dependence develop in a therapeutic context, that is, the patient finds the prescribed dose ineffective and tries higher and higher doses. Abuse occurs in a non-medical context and comprises the use, orally or intravenously, of large doses of various barbiturates, depending on their availability. Medium- and short-acting compounds such as amylobarbitone and quinalbarbitone are generally preferred to long-acting compounds such as phenobarbitone.

Barbiturates are highly dangerous in overdose, deliberate or accidental. The lethal dose is often as low as 10–20 times the anti-anxiety dose. The shorter-acting compounds are the most lethal, and alcohol is a powerful potentiator both in biochemical terms and in precipitating depression and disinhibition leading to either suicidal intent in deliberate overdoses and confusion in accidental overdoses.

Other Older Anti-anxiety Compounds

Meprobamate was introduced in the 1950s as a tranquilliser, and has muscle-relaxant as well as sedative properties. Although it was immensely popular for a while, and is still available, it was rapidly supplanted by the benzodiazepines. Its mode of action is unclear but it closely resembles the barbiturates in most respects. It is medium-acting in duration and has neurological and psychological effects and dependence and abuse liability similar to those of the barbiturates. In addition, it tends to induce rashes.

Chlormethiazole has been widely used for 30 years or so as a sedative and anticonvulsant. It also acts on the GABA-chloride complex, thereby potentiating the inhibitory effects of GABA. It is fairly short-acting with an elimination half-life of 4–6 hours in the young and 4–12 hours in the elderly. It is given by mouth to control symptoms of acute alcohol withdrawal, to manage restlessness and agitation in the elderly and as a hypnotic. Adverse reactions include sneezing, nasal congestion, irritation of the conjunctivae (whites of the eyes) and headache. Low blood-pressure can occur. Dependence may supervene on long-term use particularly in patients with prior alcohol problems. The combination of chlormethiazole and alcohol can lead to severe impairment of breathing and even death.

THE BENZODIAZEPINES

Mode of Action

The biochemical mode of action of the benzodiazepines (BZD for short) was unclear until about 15 years ago. Then it was shown that the BZDs bind to receptor sites on the inhibitory $GABA_A$-chloride complex. GABA is the most ubiquitous inhibitory neurotransmitter in the brain and spinal cord. At the $GABA_A$ sites (but not the $GABA_B$), it binds to its own receptor and increases the opening of a channel ('ionophore') across the nerve cell membrane. When the channel opens, chloride ions flow into the nerve cell altering its ionic equilibrium and making the neuron less likely to fire. Benzodiazepines potentiate this effect, thus exerting a generally depressant effect. However, unlike the barbiturates they do not have direct effects on the chloride channel.

Thus, they can only maximise normally-occurring, GABA-mediated inhibition, a factor probably accounting for their relative safety in overdose.

An almost unique property of the BZD receptor is that it can mediate three effects. At all other receptors, two effects can be mediated, the normal action on the neuron by the agonist drug, and prevention of that effect by an antagonist. For example, in a cholinergic synapse, acetylcholine (and synthetic analogues) are agonists, activating the receptor mechanisms, whereas atropine is an antagonist, blocking agonist actions. The BZD receptor has similar properties, the benzodiazepine drugs being agonist whilst flumazenil is an antagonist preventing the BZD from exerting its actions. However, in addition, the BZD receptor recognises a group of drugs, dubbed 'inverse agonists', which bind to the BZD receptor and prevent the action of GABA. They decrease chloride flow into the neuron and can increase the likelihood of anxiety and convulsions. Furthermore, intermediate compounds exist. Thus, partial agonists have been developed in the hope that these compounds will have anti-anxiety efficacy without psychomotor and cognitive effects or dependence and abuse potential.

Much is known of the detailed molecular biology of the benzodiazepine-$GABA_A$-chloride complex. It comprises five subunits and several different types of subunits exist. Theoretically, over 1000 different BZD receptors could exist but there are reasons for believing that the probable number is between 50 and 100. Various compounds are being developed with differential affinities for various subtypes of receptor, the hope being that particular BZD therapeutic functions can be targeted, e.g. anticonvulsant without sedative properties. Many fascinating possibilities have been opened by these advances in molecular pharmacology and biophysics.

Pharmacokinetics

Two aspects of BZD pharmacokinetics are of practical importance. First, the speed of onset of action depends on the mode of administration and rapidity of penetration to the brain. Thus, diazepam is effective in stopping repeated epileptic fits (status epilepticus) when given intravenously. Given this way, it is also useful, usually together with antipsychotic medication, in quietening the disturbed patient. By contrast, other BZDs (e.g. oxazepam) are less rapidly absorbed and take some time to exert a calming effect. Some BZDs redistribute rapidly from the brain to other tissues so they actually have short durations of action on single administration.

The metabolic half-lives of the BZDs vary greatly and some have important active metabolites which prolong their action. A group of drugs such as chlordiazepoxide and diazepam are long-acting both because they are fairly slowly metabolised but also give rise to a very persistent psychotropically active metabolite. In contrast oxazepam and lorazepam are medium-acting in duration and have no active metabolites. In fact, the metabolism of these latter compounds is relatively simple and is not altered in the young, the old or the physically ill. A number of studies have examined the relationship between plasma BZD concentrations and clinical response but no clinically useful conclusions have been drawn.

Pharmacology

As outlined above, BZDs potentiate the inhibitory effects of GABA on a wide range of physiological functions in the brain. BZDs can reduce the turnover of neurotransmitters such as acetylcholine, noradrenaline and 5-HT. The main sites of action of the BZDs are on the spinal cord where muscle relaxant effects are mediated, the brain-stem where they may be involved in anticonvulsant effects, the cerebellum, causing ataxia perhaps, and the limbic and cortical areas involved in the organisation of emotional experience and behaviour. These actions are reversed when the BZDs are withdrawn and 'overshoot' may occur, accounting for rebound and perhaps withdrawal syndromes.

The BZDs differ in their profile of actions. Thus, some such as clonazepam have marked anticonvulsant properties, diazepam is a powerful muscle relaxant, and lorazepam appears to affect memory functions strongly. Alprazolam (and adinazolam) have been claimed to have antidepressant properties. The reasons for these differential profiles have not been clearly established.

Clinical Uses

Studies evaluating the clinical efficacy of the BZDs run into many thousands, the main indications being insomnia (see Chapter 8), generalised anxiety, panic and most recently, social phobia and post-traumatic stress disorder. The problem of carefully defining patient groups tends to be addressed by using the American Psychiatric Association's DSM-III-R criteria. The main anxiety indication is well-established, with an apparently prompt onset of action.

The BZDs are widely used in primary care in the management of anxiety and stress-related conditions. The indications in practice are much wider than DSM-III-R GAD with its emphasis on excessive anxiety. The BZDs are used to assuage the anxieties and pangs of everyday life, fear of unemployment, marital dysharmony, and the like. As will be seen later, the problems of the BZDs have become apparent and have been widely publicised. This has resulted in a substantial reduction in the prescription of BZDs as anti-anxiety compounds (but no fall in hypnotic prescriptions).

There seems little to choose among the BZDs with respect to efficacy. The individual patient may develop a preference but this often relates to dosages not being equivalent. For example, lorazepam was regarded as five times more potent than diazepam and consequently prescribed in a fifth of the dose, e.g. 1 mg thrice daily compared with 5 mg thrice daily for diazepam. However, lorazepam is more potent than this and a more appropriate dosage would be 0.5 mg three times a day. Only recently have tablets of this strength become available.

A comprehensive programme of research has evaluated the use of high-dose alprazolam in the management of patients with panic disorder. Suppression of panics usually occurs quite promptly and there may be substantial clinical improvement. However, withdrawal of the alprazolam is usually followed by rebound panics or even a withdrawal syndrome. This is hardly surprising in view of the high doses and long treatment courses used. Some studies compared alprazolam with the TCA imipramine as well as placebo. Although early drop-out with the TCA is higher than with the BZD, the longer-term outcome is no different and discontinuing the imipramine is easier. Many practitioners prefer imipramine or clomipramine as the drug of first choice, reserving alprazolam for those who cannot tolerate a TCA.

Initially, claims were made that alprazolam had unique anti-panic properties among the BZDs. However, more recent studies have suggested that other BZDs in high doses are capable of suppressing panics.

Unwanted Effects

Some acute adverse effects relate to neurological function and are listed earlier. The unsteadiness may lead to falls, which in the elderly can result in fractured limbs. Other effects in the long-term include weight gain, rash, impairment of sexual function and menstrual disturbances. EEG changes such as increase in fast-wave activity are characteristic of the BZDs and may be used to monitor their use.

A few studies have hinted at possible neuroanatomical changes in long-term users. The changes resemble those seen in patients with alcohol-related problems and it is difficult to exclude this contaminating influence. Even if such abnormalities were confirmed, it might indicate a non-specific abnormality predisposing to long-term anxiety and BZD use, rather than a direct effect of long-term BZDs on brain structures. Further work with up-to-date sophisticated neuroimaging techniques is clearly justified.

The subjective side-effects of the BZDs are well-documented with the numerous clinical trials, many with placebo controls, giving a true estimate of drug-related adverse effects. The most common subjective complaints are drowsiness and tiredness, but dizziness and 'bursting in the head' are also complained of quite frequently. The subjective effects are most marked following the first few doses but generally wane thereafter. The severity of the symptoms depends on the dose, the sensitivity of the patient, and to a lesser extent the BZD involved, some such as diazepam being more sedative than others such as clobazam. Older patients are more sensitive than younger subjects because they metabolise many BZDs more slowly, thereby attaining higher drug levels. Also the elderly brain is more sensitive to BZDs.

'Paradoxical' responses can develop in some individuals, although it is not clear how frequent or serious such reactions are. The commonest is an increase instead of a decrease in anxiety although this may be misinterpreted as a worsening of the original anxiety. More dramatic is an increase in hostile feelings, which may rarely culminate in anti-social acts. Aggressive and irritable feelings may perplex the patient who fails to relate them to his medication. Patients with 'impulse dyscontrol' are believed to be at particular risk. Other responses include giggling, laughing or weeping, and uncharacteristic behaviour such as shop-lifting and sexual improprieties.

BZDs have been accused of causing depression in some individuals, this being regarded as a paradoxical response. The consensus is that the BZDs are not true antidepressants but can elevate mood by inducing mild euphoria. Patients with depression often have marked anxiety, which may mask the primary affect. Lessening that anxiety will render the depression more obvious. It is best to conclude that BZDs are neutral with respect to depression, neither treating it nor precipitating it.

Drug Interactions

BZDs have few interactions with other drugs at the pharmacokinetic, metabolic level. Nevertheless, marked potentiations can occur at the functional level. The best-studied is that with alcohol which can lead to greatly increased effects, both depressant and paradoxical. Modelling these interactions in the laboratory generally involves giving single doses of each: potentiation is often apparent. If, however, the BZD is given repeatedly, and then alcohol added, potentiation may not occur because tolerance to the BZD is transferred to the alcohol, lessening, not increasing its effects. Nevertheless, in practice potentiation does often occur and patients must be warned not to take alcohol when being treated with a BZD.

Overdose

Overdose with BZDs is common but a fatal outcome is rare. However, if other drugs such as alcohol or tricyclic antidepressants are taken at the same time, then death may ensue. The young, the old, and those with respiratory problems are at definite risk.

After an overdose, the person becomes drowsy or stuporose and may lapse into a light coma. A few develop rigidity or coma. Blood-pressure drops a little but respiration is hardly affected. Sleep lasts 24–48 hours and the person generally wakes naturally. However, if the diagnosis is in doubt, the benzodiazepine antagonist, flumazenil, can be injected to temporarily arouse the patient.

Dependence and Withdrawal

The BZDs were judged by doctors and patients alike to be safe and effective remedies with a negligible risk of inducing dependence. This contributed to their astonishing popularity. Lone voices challenged this perception pointing out that both animal and human studies had identified a definite dependence risk. In turn, it was pointed out by the protagonists of the BZDs that very few patients escalated their dose, a sure sign of dependence. Rather they stayed at the original therapeutic dose level over years of usage.

About 15 years ago, the widespread and long-term usage of the BZDs became an increasing concern. The possibility was mooted that these chronic users were actually physically dependent on their therapeutic dose and escalation of dose was not an essential marker for dependence. Several investigators carried out clinical studies of various types and showed that a withdrawal syndrome akin to that known to follow barbiturate use could be detected in about a third of long-term BZD users on discontinuation. Initially, many clinicians remained sceptical, attributing any recrudescence of symptoms to return of the underlying anxiety disorder. However, further studies established the presence of newly emergent symptoms on discontinuing BZDs, a cardinal feature of a withdrawal syndrome. At present the debate has shifted to questions about the frequency, severity and clinical significance of the withdrawal syndrome.

The BZD withdrawal syndrome includes symptoms of anxiety, shakiness, trembling, insomnia, impaired concentration, nausea, loss of appetite and weight, headaches, dizziness, dysphoria, lethargy and tiredness. Symptoms of perceptual hypersensitivity are particularly characteristic and include feelings of lights being too bright, sounds too loud and unsteadiness. Hot and cold flushes, muscle weakness and a general 'flu-like' feeling are also common. The withdrawal syndrome is time-locked to the discontinuation of the BZD, coming on up to 48 hours after stopping a medium-duration compound such as lorazepam, but may be delayed up to a week or so after stopping diazepam. Tapering the dose lessens but does not always obviate the withdrawal syndrome. This can be contrasted with the return of an anxiety syndrome, which is not typically time-locked to drug cessation but more to the status of external stresses.

The probability of a withdrawal syndrome depends on the duration of BZD use. Before four weeks, symptoms are rare, beyond a year more common. Dosage is important in determining the probability of a withdrawal syndrome but the severity of the syndrome is not necessarily worse after tapering off a high dose. However, some BZDs such as lorazepam and alprazolam have the reputation of being the most difficult to withdraw from, and some data from controlled studies support this clinical impression.

The natural history of BZD withdrawal is not well-studied. Most patients experience a fairly short syndrome of a few weeks, but a few have protracted reactions. Success rates vary greatly depending on the type of patient. In primary care, success is the rule but in special clinics, at least 30% fail to achieve complete abstinence. The factors governing outcome are unclear but pre-existing depression is an indicator of poor outcome, as is a 'dependent' personality or one that cannot tolerate stress. Some patients undergo prolonged withdrawal, their initial symptoms persisting for months or years. Such patients were over-represented in the several thousand litigants suing the manufacturers of BZDs.

The Management of BZD Withdrawal

The most important factor for the success of any withdrawal strategy is the patient's desire and intent to come off BZDs. Often minimal intervention consisting of encouragement, advice and support is sufficient. Patients who do not respond may need a more formal withdrawal strategy. In this case it is important to conduct a careful assessment to identify any underlying psychiatric condition such as depression or alcohol abuse. Then a schedule of withdrawal is planned with the patient (Table 7.1). This may involve the substitution of a long-acting compound and some rationalisation of drug taking to break associations at first. Then a graduated withdrawal is planned with the patient which takes place over a six to eight week period. The reduction may be more rapid at first as more problems tend to be encountered later on in the schedule. However, it is advisable for the patient to stay at the reduced dose for at least a week each time. It is important to offer constant support and telephone access. Adjunctive medication has not been found to be very effective in attenuating withdrawal symptoms but may be necessary

Table 7.1 Schedule of withdrawal from long-term benzodiazepine treatment

1. Conduct careful assessment
2. Ensure patient motivation and involvement
3. Rationalise drug taking
4. Substitute long-acting compound
5. Taper withdrawal over several weeks
6. Offer constant support
7. Consider adjunctive medication
8. Consider adjunctive psychological therapy

to combat pre-existing depression. Additional psychological treatment can be effective in helping patients to discontinue BZD treatment. Anxiety management training can help to improve self-efficacy and develop alternative coping strategies and cognitive behavioural therapy can help to identify and correct false beliefs.

High-dose Dependence

Although this is uncommon, it can occur particularly in patients who have had problems previously with other sedative drugs such as the barbiturates, or with alcohol. A withdrawal syndrome on discontinuation is almost inevitable, and tapering the dose must be instituted to avoid serious withdrawal effects such as fits or paranoid psychosis.

Abuse

In many countries, abuse of BZDs has become an increasing concern. Benzodiazepines can lead to euphoria and therefore do have some abuse liability especially when used in high doses or intravenously. It has been shown that both abstinent alcoholics and the sons of alcoholics experience more drug induced changes in euphoria to benzodiazepines and may therefore be at high risk for abuse. They are also used by multiple drug users to potentiate opioid effects and temper the effects of stopping stimulants. However, increasingly BZDs are used intravenously on their own. In the UK, the major problem involves the injection of temazepam. This hypnotic drug was originally formulated and marketed as a liquid-filled capsule, the contents of which could be easily injected. Reformulated as gel-filled capsules, the addicts found ways of liquifying the contents but subsequent injection resulted in horrendous local damage and even loss of limbs.

Psychological Effects of Benzodiazepines

Severe anxiety can have a widespread deleterious effect on performance and studies which have compared patients suffering from GAD, PD and OCD with healthy controls have consistently shown drug-free patients to be impaired on psychological tests. Thus effective anti-anxiety medication may improve performance by suppressing anxiety. However, both the severity of the disorder and the dose of the drug are important mediating factors. As the benzodiazepines are the most widely prescribed group of psychotropic drugs, they have also been the most widely investigated and so this section can only be a brief summary of the work. Most of the work has been conducted on single doses in healthy volunteers.

Effects of Benzodiazepines in Healthy Volunteers

The best known subjective effect of benzodiazepines is sedation. Despite improved specificity of action from the barbiturates and meprobamate, drowsiness or tiredness is readily apparent and can be detected on visual analogue scales acutely after each dose even after one or two weeks' administration. In contrast to the sedation produced by antipsychotics, subjects report it as a largely pleasant sensation and may experience calming or even euphoric feelings at the same time. Benzodiazepines therefore do have some abuse liability and misusers consume large doses in a way that maximises brain penetration (speed of onset) e.g. intravenous, sniffing.

Sedation can also be measured objectively in the laboratory. Early work showed psychological impairment could be measured on a variety of tasks several hours after consumption. A review of 27 studies in 1979 indicated a positive relationship between magnitude of effect and dosage level but was unable to discriminate between benzodiazepines because of the few studies comparing different compounds and the diversity of the psychomotor tests used. However, it was possible to conclude that the functions showing consistent impairment were speed of repetitive movements and acquisition of new material. There was little evidence that benzodiazepines affected visual-spatial, perceptual, verbal or arithmetical faculties and the authors concluded that there was relatively little indication at that time that well established higher mental faculties were adversely affected.

As well as acute effects, benzodiazepines have been shown to produce impairment for up to a day after use as hypnotics, even when several hours sleep have intervened. A review of 52 studies in 1982 concluded that all hypnotics produce decrements in performance the next day, the extent of this impairment being dependent on dose but not consistently on half-life. Most of the tasks used were psychomotor although some (DSST, sorting, cancellation) also had a cognitive element. The functions which showed consistent impairment were speed of performance which the authors related to sedation and CNS depression but also anterograde memory, i.e. memory for information learned after drug administration, which although a well-known and indeed useful property when benzodiazepines are used intravenously as preoperative sedatives, was not expected after oral night-time administration. Putting the results of these two reviews together, there is considerable agreement. They both found that tasks involving speed and learning were most affected and those involving coordination and spatial abilities were least affected. Other studies have found that both CFFT and saccadic eye movements are sensitive to acute doses of benzodiazepines. The results on higher functions have been further clarified by specialised reviews on memory and benzodiazepines. These have confirmed that memory for information acquired pre drug (retrograde memory) is not impaired by benzodiazepines and may even be improved acutely (retrograde facilitation) because of reduced retroactive interference from other information acquired post drug intake but that anterograde amnesia is common with all benzodiazepines. The most sensitive tasks are those of increased complexity and involving a delay in recall because more demands are made on memory. Tasks involving primary memory, nondeclarative memory or retrieval from secondary semantic memory generally show little impairment although performance may be slowed.

There is some evidence that tolerance develops to the sedative effects of benzodiazepines after one or two weeks of continuous administration. This has been clearly shown with saccadic eye movements. However, because of the few studies completed with more than one or two weeks treatment using therapeutic doses, in which clear tolerance has been shown, this widely held belief is difficult to substantiate with more complex or cognitive tasks. In fact there is some evidence that tolerance to memory decrements does not develop in this time.

Effects of Benzodiazepines in Patients

There are too few studies in patient populations to determine if their responses differ greatly from controls. It is evident from the review on hypnotics that insomniacs do not differ from controls in their effects on performance and there is some evidence that similar functions are affected in patients with both GAD and PD. However, patients seem to be less sensitive to these effects and require three times as much drug to obtain similar effects. As high doses are used in the treatment of PD, such effects should be easier to detect and one recent study has shown some impairment still present after eight weeks' treatment. Another approach is to test long-term users before and after withdrawal of their medication. A few studies have attempted to do this and have generally found some improvement after withdrawal.

Risk of Accidents

It has been suggested that the use of benzodiazepines contributes to an increased risk of accidents both on the road and elsewhere. Formal studies of the risk of road accidents have approached the problem from two different angles. On the one hand, numerous laboratory tasks of simulated driving and even real driving tasks both under controlled conditions named 'closed course' and in real traffic in a specially monitored car have been developed. On the other hand, epidemiological investigations have concentrated on implying drug intake from self-report or prescription monitoring or more scientifically from measuring benzodiazepine levels in the body fluids of people involved in accidents. Generally, benzodiazepines have been shown to adversely affect both simulated driving performance and actual driving ability. These methods have been criticised as not analogous to 'real' driving but some agreement has been shown between the different methods.

One prospective epidemiological study carried out in the UK estimated the relative risk of an accident in which injury or death occurred to be 4.9 times greater when 'tranquillisers' were deemed (by prescription) to be present. However, epidemiological studies also suffer from many uncontrolled variables. Firstly, psychiatric or medical patients may be at increased risk for accidents regardless of whether or not they are taking medication. Secondly, the fact that drugs were prescribed does not mean they were being taken at the time of the accident. Thirdly, even if drugs can be detected this does not mean that they were behaviourally active at the time of the accident and fourthly, the presence of other substances including alcohol is frequently a complicating factor. This means that a causal relationship can seldom be assumed. Epidemiological studies have found a frequency of benzodiazepine use ranging from 0.8–20% but those studies which have attempted most control and used a reference group, who were driving at similar locations and times at which accidents occurred, have not consistently demonstrated that benzodiazepine users are overrepresented either in the population of arrested drivers or of those involved in road traffic accidents whether fatal or not.

A few studies have attempted to examine the incidence of benzodiazepine use in other types of accident. One study of accident and injury-related health care utilisation in the USA did find that benzodiazepine users were significantly more likely to experience an accident, estimated from their use of accident-related health care, than non-users but they were also more likely to use non-accident-related health care which means that this group may just be more likely to use any sort of health care facilities more which presumably includes benzodiazepines. There is thus little evidence to implicate their use as causal in industrial accidents. However, there is some evidence that the elderly may be more prone to fall while receiving such medication although this may not result in increased bone fractures. The latter study was based on interview data but another study of hospitalised patients found no difference in falls in younger patients but confirmed that patients over 70 years old who fell were more likely to have received a prescription for a benzodiazepine. Benzodiazepines have also been implicated in drug-associated hospital admissions.

Benzodiazepine-like Compounds

A variety of compounds act on or close to the BZD receptor. The assumption was made that some at least might combine equal or even enhanced BZD-type efficacy with fewer and less severe side-effects and less propensity to induce dependence and abuse. Some are partial agonists, some selective on subtypes of BZD receptors, and others are different in an unclear way. Only one, alpidem, reached the market (in France) and preliminary data suggested that it fulfilled some at least of the above assumptions. Unfortunately, it had adverse effects on the liver and had to be withdrawn. Its analogue, zolpidem, is available as an hypnotic (see p. 120).

BUSPIRONE

Buspirone is an azapirone derivative, chemically distinct from the BZDs. Furthermore, it does not bind to the GABA-chloride complex. It does, however, bind to a subgroup of 5-HT receptors, acting as a partial agonist at 5-HT_{1A} sites. The details of the ensuing effects are ill-understood but the end result is to lessen 5-HT activity in some regions concerned with the mediation of anxiety. That the situation is even more complicated is witnessed by the fact that in higher doses buspirone appears to have full antidepressant properties.

Buspirone is used to treat anxiety but it lacks hypnotic, muscle relaxant and anticonvulsant properties. Although licensed for the short-term treatment of generalised anxiety disorder, it is often, for reasons rehearsed below, prescribed long-term for chronic anxiety disorders.

In normal clinical doses, effects on psychomotor and cognitive activity are minimal, both in normal volunteers and in patients. No interaction with alcohol is demonstrable. In clinical trials, buspirone is both equi-effective and equi-potent with diazepam but some differences are important. The onset of action of buspirone is slower than with a BZD, rather in the manner of an antidepressant. Another problem is the influence of previous BZD treatment: patients with no such prior experience respond well to buspirone whereas patients who have taken a lot of BZDs do poorly, and may have unwanted effects such as restlessness.

Although buspirone generally has fewer side-effects than a BZD, they may necessitate stopping the drug in at least 10% of patients. Starting with a low dose (say 5 mg twice-daily) and slowly increasing it minimises this risk. The commonest adverse effects are dizziness, headache, nausea, sleeplessness, and fatigue. Sedation is uncommon. The elderly tolerate buspirone well.

Particular attention has been paid to possible induction of dependence and the risk of abuse. In comparative long-term studies, stopping buspirone was routinely uneventful whereas stopping BZD treatment was followed by withdrawal problems. Buspirone is not cross-dependent with the BZDs, cannot substitute for them and does not help in the management of BZD withdrawal. Reports of abuse of buspirone have been sporadic and unconvincing but continuous monitoring in the UK and elsewhere continues. Buspirone seems as safe in overdose as a typical BZD.

Other $5\text{-}HT_{1A}$ partial agonists are in development and have shown the expected anxiolytic efficacy. Other drugs acting on 5-HT systems are also being investigated and include $5\text{-}HT_2$ and $5\text{-}HT_3$ antagonists. Other developments include the study of cholecystokinin and other neuropeptides in mediating anxiety so that further classes of drugs may eventually be developed.

Other Anxiolytic Agents

Beta-adrenoceptor antagonists ('beta-blockers') have long been used to treat anxiety, particularly in patients with bodily symptoms such as palpitations, tremor and gastro-intestinal upset. Patients with performance anxiety do particularly well. However, whether a patient obtains relief depends on the significance of that bodily symptom to the maintenance of the anxiety disorder. If the symptom is pivotal, the patient will be helped by having it blocked; if it is not crucial, then the anxiety will hardly be affected.

Other drugs used in the management of anxiety are the tricyclic antidepressants, selective serotonin re-uptake inhibitors and the monoamine oxidase inhibitors. Many of these drugs are favoured by psychiatrists for the treatment of patients with chronic anxiety, in view of fears of the dependence potential of the BZDs. Some of the newer antidepressants are being evaluated in anxiety disorders such as panic disorder, social phobia, and post-traumatic stress disorder. Efficacy is being established in all of these indications.

PSYCHOLOGICAL THERAPY OF ANXIETY DISORDERS

Drug treatment is probably most controversial in the treatment of anxiety because of the overprescription of BZDs. Most patients suffering from anxiety are treated in primary care and many episodes of anxiety or stress reactions are not prolonged and resolve spontaneously. Psychological treatments for anxiety abound and there is a vast literature dealing with them; so the following can only be a brief summary.

Counselling

Often a single counselling session, consisting of an explanation of the causes and symptoms of anxiety, reassurance about recovery and encouragement to deal with any particular problems, conducted by the GP will suffice. This initial consultation is very important in modifying the patient's view of the condition and their own role in its management and so bland reassurance may be unhelpful. In more persistent anxiety, there is evidence that problem-solving approaches (directive counselling) are helpful and studies of brief interventions using structured steps to identify problems, define the goals of treatment and ways in which to achieve these have been shown to be more effective than standard treatment which was determined by the GP and which may or may not have included medication. In severe anxiety other structured psychological approaches have been shown to be effective.

Behaviour therapy

The first behavioural treatment to be used in treating phobias was *systematic desensitisation* in which the patient is first taught a muscle relaxation technique and then asked to imagine feared stimuli according to a hierarchy previously agreed with the therapist. Anxiety must be reduced at each stage before moving on to the next. This approach has largely been replaced by *graded exposure* which involves actual rather than imaginal exposure to the feared object and does not necessitate relaxation. Graded exposure has become the established psychological treatment for both agoraphobia and OCD in which it is combined with *response prevention*. It has been shown to be as effective as drug treatment with both TCAs and BZDs and to produce more lasting effects in both disorders. Behavioural techniques such as *social skills* and *assertiveness training* have been used with patients who have problems in social functioning whatever the diagnosis. These techniques are often combined with modelling and/or role play. They have not, however, been systematically compared to drug treatment.

Cognitive Behaviour Therapy (CBT)

Over the last 25 years, there has been an increasing emphasis on the cognitive mechanisms that mediate behaviour and this has led to a growth in cognitive behavioural treatments. In social phobia, social skills are not usually impaired but social interactions tend to be viewed as potentially dangerous or shameful. In this case CBT has been shown to be comparable to treatment with both phenelzine and alprazolam and to show less relapse at six months/ one year follow-ups. In less specific disorders, like GAD, a compilation of techniques referred to as *anxiety management* has been shown to be effective. It comprises both behavioural and cognitive techniques, e.g. relaxation, mental distraction, identification and control of upsetting thoughts and graded practice in avoided activities. It may be the cognitive element, which is important in this therapy as CBT alone has been found to be as, if not more, effective. The specificity of CBT itself has also been questioned by studies finding equivalent short-term response with other forms of psychological therapy in anxiety disorders. However, CBT has been found to be equivalent to diazepam in the treatment of GAD and patients assigned to CBT had the lowest incidence of subsequent treatment intervention. CB treatments have also produced favourable results in PD without avoidance. It is important to note that key features of CBT may differ. Some authors have emphasised the importance of *respiratory control* or *paradoxical intention* as key features in the treatment package. Studies have shown CBT to be as effective as alprazolam or TCA treatment in PD. Although *applied relaxation* also reduces the incidence of panic attacks, it is less effective than CBT or imipramine on several measures. Because of the multi-faceted nature of the disorder, psychological therapy of PTSD has tended to involve packages of therapeutic techniques similar to anxiety management or *stress innoculation training*. Drugs may be used as part of this package but there are no systematic studies comparing psychological and drug treatment.

Combination of Drug Treatment with Behaviour Therapy

Few studies have compared the efficacy of drug and psychological treatments in anxiety disorders and even fewer have examined the effects of combining the treatments; so any conclusions must be tentative. Although TCAs alone have been shown to be effective in agoraphobia and panic disorder, studies are usually confounded by self-directed exposure instructions which can be a powerful treatment in their own right. Studies examining the combination have found imipramine combined with structured exposure more effective than imipramine alone but with only minor advantages over exposure alone. The very limited data with other antidepressants is consistent with the findings for imipramine. One study which examined the combination of fluvoxamine with exposure therapy in OCD found that the combination was synergistic in acute treatment with greater improvement on rituals at two months and depression at six months. However these advantages had disappeared by one year post treatment when only the advantages of exposure were shown. Studies which have looked at the combination of benzodiazepines and exposure treatment have found rather similar results. Both high dose alprazolam and low dose diazepam combined with exposure marginally enhanced gains with the single therapies during treatment but this improvement was not only lost on drug discontinuation but there was some evidence that withdrawal of alprazolam impaired the continued therapeutic gains shown on exposure alone.

Combination of Drug Treatment With Cognitive Behaviour Therapy

Studies of this combination are just starting to be published. Imipramine has been shown to have an additive effect with CBT in the acute treatment of PD. Diazepam also appears to enhance CBT as GAD patients on the combination not only showed improvement early in treatment but also showed most clinically significant change at the end of the study. In contrast to the results with exposure therapy, patients on the combination maintained initial treatment gains at six months follow-up in the same way as those on CBT alone. This result is similar to the effects of TCAs and CBT in depression and suggests that low dose benzodiazepines administered over a short time period (six to nine weeks) do not interfere with cognitive behavioural therapies. In fact as indicated earlier two studies have found that CBT may help PD patients to withdraw from benzodiazepine treatment. There are very few studies of newer anxiolytics but one has found buspirone to enhance CBT effects on generalised anxiety and agoraphobia in patients with PD with agoraphobia and improvement was maintained at one year follow-up.

SUMMARY

Benzodiazepines are effective drugs in the short-term treatment of anxiety. Long-term use should be avoided because of the possibility of dependence leading to withdrawal problems. Buspirone is a newer anti-anxiety drug but increasingly antidepressants are being used and have shown some efficacy particularly in panic disorder and obsessive-compulsive disorder. Numerous psychological therapies are used to treat anxiety. Structured approaches such as directive counselling, graded exposure and cognitive behaviour therapy are most effective. There are too few studies to evaluate the combination of drug and psychological treatment but short-term drug use does not appear to interfere with cognitive behavioural therapy.

FURTHER READING

Ashton, H. (1986) Guidelines for the rational use of benzodiazepines. When and what to use. *Drugs* **48**, 25–40.

Barlow, D.H. (1988) *Anxiety and its Disorders: The Nature and Treatment of Anxiety and Panic*. Guilford, New York.

Beck, A.T., Emery, G. and Greenberg, R.L. (1985) *Anxiety Disorders and Phobias*. Basic Books, New York.

Burrows, G.D., Judd, F.K. and Norman, T.R. (1994) Differential diagnosis and drug treatment of panic disorder, anxiety and depression. *CNS Drugs* **1**, 119–131.

Catalan, J., Gath, D.H., Anastasiades, P., Bond, S.A.K., Day, A. and Hall, L. (1991) Evaluation of a brief psychological treatment for emotional disorders in primary care. *Psychological Medicine* **21**, 1013–1018.

Choy, T. and de Bosset, F. (1992) Post-traumatic stress disorder: an overview. *Canadian Journal of Psychiatry* **37**, 578–583.

Curran, H.V. (1986) Tranquillising memories: a review of the effects of benzodiazepines on human memory. *Biological Psychology* **23**, 179–213.

Curran, H.V. (1991) Benzodiazepines, memory and mood: a review. *Psychopharmacology* **105**, 1–8.

Da Roza Davis, J. and Gelder, M. (1991) Long-term management of anxiety states. *International Review of Psychiatry* **3**, 5–17.

Deakin, J.F.W. (1993) A review of clinical efficacy of 5-HT$_{1A}$ agonists in anxiety and depression. *Journal of Psychopharmacology* **7**, 283–289.

Ghoneim, M.M. and Mewaldt, S.P. (1990) Benzodiazepines and human memory: a review. *Anesthesiology* **72**, 926–938.

Hallström, C. (ed.) (1993) *Benzodiazepine Dependence*. Oxford University Press, Oxford.

Jenike, M.A., Baer, L. and Minichiello, W.E. (eds) (1990) *Obsessive-Compulsive Disorders: Theory and Management, Second Edition*. Mosby Year Book, London.

Lister, R.G. (1985) The amnesic action of benzodiazepines in man. *Neuroscience & Biobehavioral Reviews* **9**, 87–94.

Marks, I.M. (1987) *Fears, Phobias and Rituals*. Oxford University Press, New York.

Marks, I. and O'Sullivan, G. (1988) Drugs and psychological treatments for agoraphobia/panic and obsessive-compulsive disorders: A review. *British Journal of Psychiatry* **153**, 650–658.

Michelson, L. and Ascher, L.M. (eds.) (1987) *Anxiety and Stress Disorders: Cognitive-behavioral Assessment and Treatment*. Guilford Press, New York.

Middleton, H.C. (1991) Psychology and pharmacology in the treatment of anxiety disorders: cooperation or confrontation. *Journal of Psychopharmacology* **5**, 281–285.

Morgan, J and Tyrer, P. (1994) Treating the somatic symptoms of anxiety. *CNS Drugs* **1**, 427–434.

Roy-Byrne, P.P., Cowley, D.S., Greenblatt, D.J., Shader, R.I. and Hommer, D. (1990) Reduced benzodiazepine sensitivity in panic disorder. *Archives of General Psychiatry* **47**, 534–538.

Walker, J.R., Norton, G.R. and Ross, C.A. (eds) (1991) *Panic Disorder and Agoraphobia*. Brooks/Cole Publishing Company, California.

Woods, J.H., Katz, J.L. and Winger, G. (1987) Abuse liability of benzodiazepines. *Pharmacological Reviews* **39**, 251–413.

Zohar, J., Zohar-Kadouch, R.C. and Kindler, S. (1992) Current concepts in the pharmacological treatment of obsessive-compulsive disorder. *Drugs* **43**, 210–218.

Please also see Further Reading for Chapter 6.

Chapter 8

TREATMENT OF SLEEP DISORDERS

In this chapter we describe the characteristics of normal sleep, the possible causes of both insomnia and hypersomnia and the treatments. Sleep hygiene advice, behaviour and cognitive therapies and hypnotic drugs are all discussed.

It is estimated that about a third of people who visit their general practitioners and about two-thirds of those who see psychiatrists complain of dissatisfaction with the restorative quality of their sleep. Indeed, about 5% of all general practice consultations are concerned primarily with complaints of insomnia. The elderly are particularly likely to seek help for this symptom.

Benzodiazepines are widely prescribed for this indication and, despite increasing concern about their side-effects and withdrawal problems, this usage remains high. For example, among 1020 elderly people living at home, 166 (16%) reported using hypnotic medication. Most of these users (73%) had taken their drugs for a year or more, 25% reporting drug use for more than 10 years.

The introduction of sleep laboratory recordings about 50 years ago and refinements in EEG technology has provided an 'objective' measure of sleep patterns which has contributed greatly to our understanding of sleep and also provided us with a powerful tool to investigate people with sleep complaints. It also furnishes us with very detailed information about drug effects. Thus, the hypnotic effects of various benzodiazepines have been evaluated in coruscating detail, allowing comprehensive comparisons, in a manner unknown with their use as anxiolytics, muscle relaxants, or even anticonvulsants. It is therefore essential to first outline what is known about normal and abnormal sleep 'architecture'.

THE CHARACTERISTICS OF NORMAL SLEEP

Sound sleep is generally regarded to involve:

1. less than half an hour to fall asleep,

2. six to eight hours of sleep with two or fewer brief awakenings,
3. a well-rested and refreshed feeling the next day.

However, over half of people complaining of poor sleep show a 'normal' sleep pattern in the laboratory suggesting that the restorative process implicit in sound sleep depends strongly on subjective factors.

The 24 hour daily rhythm (circadian) is strongly established in most people. Before falling asleep, body temperature and metabolism and cortisol production all diminish. This continues for the first half of the night but then reverses. Sleeping in the evening has an unfavourable effect on the ensuing night's sleep.

All-night polysomnograms have distinguished two main sleep states (Figure 8.1):

A. Non-rapid eye movement sleep (non-REM, orthodox sleep), itself sub-divided into four levels:

Stage 1:   The EEG comprises low-voltage desynchronised activity.
Stage 2:   Frequent 13–15 Hz trains of waves — the sleep 'spindles', often also high-voltage spikes, so-called 'K-complexes'.
Stage 3:   Delta waves, high voltage slow-activity occurring in bursts.
Stage 4:   Dominated by delta activity.

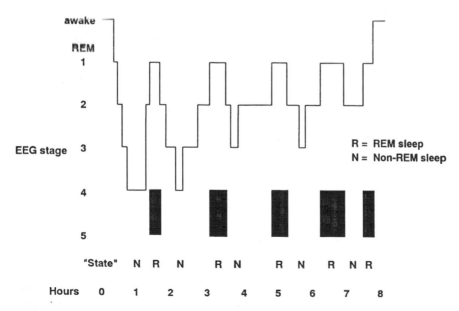

Figure 8.1   Sleep stages in a young adult

The latter two stages are often combined into one stage, 'slow-wave-sleep' (SWS). Eye movements are infrequent in non-REM sleep, bodily functions are quiescent and dreaming not typical.

B. Rapid eye movement sleep (REM) or paradoxical sleep, characterised by bursts of rapid conjugate eye movements accompanied by low voltage EEG waves. The musculature is relaxed but autonomic activity is considerable with rapid heart beat, sweating and penile erection in the male. A dream is usually reported if the subject is awakened during this phase.

The sleep period generally divides into four or five cycles per night. Each starts with NREM sleep and ends with a period of REM sleep, the cycle duration being about 90 minutes. Deep sleep (SWS) is most apparent in the earlier cycles, stages 1, 2 and REM sleep dominating the later cycles. NREM stages 1 and 2 comprise about 50% of total sleep time, SWS about 20%, and REM about 25%. The remaining 5% or so is spent transiently awake. However, the elderly have much lower voltage SWS, and total sleep time is reduced, with frequent awakenings.

Insomnia is a subjective complaint and the appraisal of the previous night's sleep as good or bad is dependent not only on sleep latency and total sleep time but also on the number of awakenings and the total pattern of sleep. The early part of the night is particularly important, the second half being regarded as optional sleep. This lessens with increasing age and is more sensitive to disturbance in general. Sleep recordings help establish the pattern of sleep although it must be remembered that many insomniacs have very variable sleep from night to night. Quite often poor nights and better nights alternate.

Several brain mechanisms are involved in sleep. The reticular formation in the pons is important in generating REM sleep and acts in opposition to serotonergic cells in the dorsal raphe nuclei. Lesioning of noradrenergic tracts results in hypersomnia. Cholinergic pathways are involved in both sleep and waking.

INSOMNIA

Insomnia is a subjective complaint of too much wakefulness. Clinically, there are three main types, difficulty in initiating sleep (DIS), difficulty maintaining sleep (DMS) and both together (DIMS). All are associated with feelings of tiredness the next day. In general practice, complaints of insomnia become significant when they last for more than three weeks and involve four or more nights per week. By this time, a negative conditioning process sets in so the patient becomes averse to going to bed fearing he or she will not sleep. There are many possible causes (Table 8.1). Healthy people often have bouts of

Table 8.1   Causes of insomnia

Cause	Examples
Acute situational stress	Jet lag
	Shift work
On-going personal stress	Bereavement
	Unemployment
Psychiatric illness	Anxiety
	Depression
Primary sleep disorder	Sleep apnoea
	Nocturnal myoclonus
Behavioural	Poor sleep hygiene

sleeplessness at times of mental and physical stress but occasionally for no apparent reason. Such 'spontaneous' insomnia may show some cyclical patterns and may represent a subclinical affective disorder. However, it is important to acknowledge that some people are constitutionally poor sleepers with delayed, shortened and fragmented sleep patterns.

Good sleep does not necessarily equate to long duration of sleep. Short sleepers can awake feeling perfectly refreshed and have sleep patterns with proportionately more SWS and less REM. Some fortunate people are quite happy and function well on only five hours sleep per night, others feel exhausted after nine hours sleep.

Insomnia is generally divided into:

1. transient insomnia associated with stress or jet-lag,
2. short-term insomnia associated with a longer-term stress reaction,
3. long-term insomnia with multifarious causes.

Transient insomnia due to jet-lag is now quite a common experience. A short-acting benzodiazepine may be quite effective in combating insomnia while the individual readjusts. Melatonin may also help.

Careful history-taking is essential and it may help for the patient to keep a sleep diary (Figure 8.2). In about half of cases, anxiety and stress underlie the difficulty in sleeping. The severity of the sleep disturbance reflects the impact of the stress on the person: he/she takes his/her problems to bed with him/her, ruminating over the sources of the stress but often not in a constructive way. As time slips by, he/she becomes more and more anxious, worrying that he/she will feel tired the next day and even more ill-equipped to cope. A vicious circle is entrained.

Sleep Diary
(to be completed each morning)

1. What time did you try to go to sleep?   _____

2. How long did it take you to fall asleep?   _____

3. Did you wake up during the night?   YES/NO
    If yes,   How many times?   _____
                How long did you stay
                awake each time?   _____

4. Do you remember dreaming?   YES/NO
    If yes, Did you have any unpleasant dreams?   YES/NO

5. What time did you wake up this morning?   _____

6. How did you feel when you woke up?
    Sleepy _____ Alert

7. What was the quality of your sleep?
    Good _____ Bad

8. What time did you actually get up?   _____

Figure 8.2   Example of a sleep diary

More severe psychiatric disorders associated with insomnia include affective disorders, anxiety disorders, schizophrenia and dementia. Total sleep time is reduced in most patients in these categories, and sleep latency is prolonged. SWS is reduced in depressive disorders. REM sleep is disrupted in various ways in most of the above disorders, with latency to the first REM period often being substantially reduced. The onset of dementia in the elderly is often accompanied by insomnia and increasing disruption of sleep patterns, culminating in reversal of the sleep pattern.

In many physical illnesses sleep may be disturbed because of a troublesome symptom. These include pain, cough, itching, indigestion, breathlessness, and reflux oesophagitis. Often a symptom can be borne in the day but becomes distracting at night. The treatment of insomnia of this type is essentially that of the distressful symptom. However, hypnotics are certainly indicated if necessary, particularly in terminal conditions where the risk of dependence is irrelevant. Nevertheless, careful prescribing is essential to avoid unfortunate complications such as respiratory depression leading to bronchopneumonia.

A wide range of drugs may induce insomnia. The common condition of rebound insomnia on discontinuation of an hypnotic medication is discussed later. Stimulant compounds can disrupt sleep, particularly sympathomimetic amines, ephedrine and the amphetamines. Some psychotropic drugs like pimozide and the SSRIs may interfere with sleep. Alcohol is a general cerebral depressant and as such induces sleep. However, it is metabolised quite rapidly and so this effect declines after a few hours. Although low doses are unlikely to disrupt sleep, the effects of larger amounts generally wear off by the middle of the night and the rest of the night's sleep is disturbed by rebound insomnia. Caffeine is also disruptive of sleep despite claims to the contrary: polysomnographic studies show a poorer quality of sleep following a caffeinated drink at bedtime than a decaffeinated one. Small amounts of nicotine are unlikely to affect sleep but smoking just before retiring to bed may delay sleep onset. The average smoker sleeps about 30 mins less than a non-smoker.

Several specific causes of insomnia have been described. The most serious is the *sleep apnoea syndrome* which usually occurs in overweight men with some upper respiratory airway obstruction. As the pharyngeal muscles relax during sleep, the obstruction increases and the sufferer struggles for breath, waking transiently. The patient feels tired the next day but is often unaware of the frequent arousals. The bed-partner usually gives a graphic account of horrendous snoring alternating with cessation of breathing.

Another condition is the 'periodic leg movement syndrome' ('restless legs') in which repetitive contractions of the legs occur. *Nocturnal myoclonus* comprises jerking of the limbs which can occur at any stage of sleep. Benzodiazepines can help both restless legs and myoclonus, which are probably related syndromes. However, they are contraindicated in sleep apnoea because they may depress respiration even further.

Finally, in as many as 20% of patients presenting with the complaint of insomnia, no cause can be convincingly established.

SLEEP HYGIENE

Recently, it has become widely accepted that hypnotic drugs should not be the mainstay of the treatment of sleep disorders. The first line of treatment should therefore be a nonpharmacological approach and should begin with the taking of an adequate history. Patients with short-lived problems or acute disturbances may then respond to relatively simple advice and procedures. The pattern and length of sleep is not uniform, yet many people have false expectations of the sleep they need, especially as they get older. People not only need less sleep as they age but they experience decreases in periods of deep or delta wave sleep and increases in light sleep which results in more night-time awakenings. However, the elderly also spend more time in bed resulting in a decreased sleep efficiency index (i.e. total sleep time divided by total time in bed). An important aspect of sleep hygiene is to have a realistic expectation of sleep.

Some people, particularly the young, can sleep well under virtually all circumstances. However, as age or other factors intervene, sleep may become disrupted and the environment becomes increasingly important. Providing oneself with an ideal set of sleep circumstances is known as practising good sleep hygiene. Many attempts have been made to isolate factors that may cause or contribute to problems with sleep and researchers agree on most of these (Table 8.2) although there are wide individual differences. The physical environment including the bed is of course extremely important. Excessively hard surfaces may cause more body movements and a lighter level of sleep with more awakenings but personal preference is paramount. Partners may interfere with each other's sleep but the absence of the habitual physical presence of a loved one may also disrupt sleep. It is better to avoid extremes of temperature, either heat or cold. It has been found that when the temperature goes above 75°F people wake more frequently, move about more, sleep less deeply and have less REM sleep. However when the temperature is very low, sleep onset may be delayed. Gentle familiar noise or low music may be soothing and help induce sleep but louder noise, especially if sporadic can be very disruptive. Sensitivity to noise varies considerably but anxious people and the elderly are generally more affected.

The common substances which interfere with sleep have already been outlined. Although people may realise that coffee affects their sleep, they may not know that caffeine is present in numerous other beverages and medicines which they may unwittingly take to promote sleep, e.g. chocolate or pain-killers.

Table 8.2   Factors affecting sleep

Factor	Good hygiene
Physical environment	
temperature	Avoid extreme heat/cold
noise	Avoid sporadic loud noises
	Use soothing music
Sleep interfering substances	Avoid caffeine, nicotine, alcohol
	Take a warm, milky drink
Sleep scheduling pattern	Establish a regular pattern
	Avoid daytime naps
Pre-sleep activities	Avoid exercise, activity, worry
	Indulge in relaxation, reading, warm bath
Daytime behaviour	Regular exercise
	Good diet

It is important to try to maintain a regular pattern of sleep, attempting to go to bed and rise at a similar time each day. Sleeping late at the weekend may delay sleep in the evening and lead to tiredness on Monday morning. The insomnia sufferer may develop an irregular pattern of sleeping across the entire week. Attempts to make up sleep by going to bed very early or napping during the day usually cause disruption of the sleep-wake rhythm leading to more problems.

The time just before going to bed serves as a transition period between waking and sleep. It is a time for relaxation and winding-down from daytime activities. The development of a set of pre-bedtime routines each night can be helpful. While this is usually recognised and practised for children in the form of baths and bedtime stories, it is often neglected by adults.

Daytime behaviour influences the quality and quantity of sleep. Taking regular exercise is conducive to deeper, restorative sleep and this is best taken in the late afternoon or early evening. Occasional exercise does not have the same beneficial effect and exercise late in the evening is likely to delay sleep onset and should be avoided. Weight loss or taking insufficient calories, whether deliberately or accidentally, is likely to disrupt sleep. The intake of food then usually assists sleep and a light snack or milky drink may be beneficial. It is not advisable to eat heavy meals just before retiring because this will stimulate digestive activity which can interfere with sleep.

It is important that people with sleep difficulties are educated not only in the knowledge but in the practice of sleep hygiene as there is some evidence that although poor sleepers have more knowledge than good sleepers, they practise it less often. It is hard to know which comes first, poor sleep or poor sleep hygiene but it is important to intervene in the vicious circle.

Good sleep hygiene advice may be all that is necessary for patients with mild to moderate sleep disturbance or short-term problems but those with more severe or chronic sleep disorders or who have become dependent on hypnotics will need more structured psychological treatment.

PSYCHOLOGICAL TREATMENT

Psychological treatment should always be preceded by detailed assessment. Many procedures exist including structured interviews and questionnaires but a daily sleep diary (Figure 8.2) is generally invaluable in isolating specific problems. There are various therapeutic approaches (Table 8.3) and these will be only briefly described as other texts cover them comprehensively.

Progressive muscular relaxation is probably the technique which has been used

Table 8.3   Psychological treatments for sleep disorders

Progressive muscular relaxation
Autogenic training
Stimulus control
Sleep restriction
Chronotherapy
Cognitive therapy

most widely. The patient is taught to contract and relax groups of muscles throughout the body, thus enabling him/her to identify moderate levels of tension and to be able to relieve this. While relaxation is targeted at the body, *autogenic training* is a mental exercise in which the subject repeats self-suggestions of heaviness and warmth. Both these techniques have been shown to improve problems with sleep onset.

Sleep can be considered as a stimulus controlled behaviour in that it usually takes place in a specific setting, e.g. in bed at night. *Stimulus control treatment* then aims to identify weaknesses which have developed in the stimulus and to reinforce the strength of environmental events which serve as signals for sleep. Patients are therefore encouraged to only go to bed when drowsy, to avoid activities not associated with sleep in the bedroom and to get up if sleep does not ensue after a certain period of time. Instructions are given and practice records completed. Many patients find that sleep is delayed because of worrying about daytime activities and then eventually by the worry of not being able to fall asleep. The behavioural treatment for this is to set aside a definite time of day to do this kind of worrying and to prepare for the next day, which is not within an hour of bedtime. The cognitive behavioural approach is to use *paradoxical intention* in which the patient engages deliberately in the feared behaviour and attempts to stay awake. More recently *cognitive therapy* has embraced this form of sleep problem by encouraging patients to recognise and challenge pre-sleep ruminations and replace them with rational alternatives.

Sleep restriction is another behavioural technique which aims to improve the sleep efficiency index. Clients are encouraged to restrict the time they spend in bed to the number of hours they usually sleep. They may experience some sleep deprivation initially due to their underestimation of actual sleep time but they are then allowed to gradually increase the time spent in bed until a satisfactory sleep efficiency index is obtained.

Most people only realise that their sleep is strongly influenced by circadian rhythms when they have to sleep at an unusual time of day due to shift work or travel to a different time zone. Some people, however, exhibit 'delayed sleep phase syndrome', i.e. they are unable to fall asleep until 4 or 5 a.m. but then sleep well. *Chronotherapy* is used to reset their internal clock. As it is easier to move this forwards than backwards, bedtime is delayed by three hours a day until sleep onset coincides with the desired bedtime.

A recent meta-analysis of psychological treatments for insomnia found that five hours of (weekly) therapy produced reliable and persistent changes in sleep onset and time awake after onset. Sleep hygiene education was not sufficient to produce significant improvement alone but was usually incorporated into multicomponent interventions. Focused therapies like stimulus control and sleep restriction were the most effective procedures.

The important factor in all these treatments is firstly to correct misperceptions and then to increase the patients' control over sleep and thereby their feeling of self-efficacy. The occasional use of an hypnotic is unlikely to threaten this and may help to reinforce the sleep-wake cycle. However, daily use should be avoided.

HYPNOTIC DRUGS

Many drugs are used to treat insomnia symptomatically, including benzodiazepines and the barbiturates. Newer classes comprise cyclopyrrolone derivatives such as zopiclone and imidazopyridines like zolpidem. However, a range of other compounds are still used such as chloral derivatives, chlormethiazole, antihistamines, sedative antidepressants and antipsychotics. The choice of an hypnotic agent takes into account factors such as efficacy, rapidity of onset of action, safety, minimal daytime residual sedation and lack of rebound on discontinuation. The shorter-acting benzodiazepines (see Chapter 7) meet most but not all of these requirements and in most countries are the most frequently used hypnotic agents. Adverse effects such as daytime sedation, neuropsychiatric reactions (amnesia, depression) and rebound are strongly dose-dependent. Clinical and regulatory pressures have tended in the direction of increasingly conservative treatment regimens, with respect of dosage, duration of treatment and intermittency of administration.

About 10 benzodiazepines are widely-used worldwide. They divide into the long-, medium- and short-acting compounds (Table 8.4). By and large, these drugs are quite quickly absorbed and penetrate rapidly to the brain. Hence their primary therapeutic effect is to shorten time to sleep onset. They also 'consolidate' sleep (fewer awakenings and transitions across sleep stages) but usually in the first half of the night. Prolongation of total sleep time is not consistently achieved, even by the long-acting compounds. Benzodiazepine

Table 8.4   Dosage, half-life and duration of some hypnotic drugs used in the treatment of insomnia

Drug	Dosage (mg)	$t_{\frac{1}{2}}$ (h)	Duration
Benzodiazepines			
Estazolam	1–2	8–24	Intermediate
Flunitrazepam	0.5–1	10–20	Intermediate
Flurazepam	15–30	48–120	Long
Loprazolam	1–2	4–11	Intermediate
Lormetazepam	1–2	8–11	Intermediate
Nitrazepam	5–10	25–35	Long
Quazepam	7.5–15	48–120	Long
Temazepam	15–30	8–20	Intermediate
Triazolam	0.125–0.25	2–6	Short
Nonbenzodiazepines			
Zolpidem	10–20	1.5–2.5	Short
Zopiclone	7.5–15	5–6	Short

hypnotics typically reduce slow-wave sleep and REM sleep, and prolong the time to the first REM episode.

Zopiclone and zolpidem are chemically non-benzodiazepine but share many pharmacological properties. Both are short-acting and almost devoid of residual daytime sedation in low dose. It is not yet clear whether rebound and dependence are less likely to occur with these compounds than with similar benzodiazepines given in equivalent dosage. Zolpidem in particular has little effect on sleep architecture.

Chloral derivatives are still popular but can cause gastric irritation and rashes. High-dose dependence is a definite risk and chloral is dangerous in overdosage. Chlormethiazole has a brief duration of action but is dependence-inducing and can cause confusion, especially in the elderly.

Antihistamines are often used to sedate children but are long-acting and dangerous in overdosage. Antidepressants are being used as hypnotics because of concerns over the benzodiazepines. Trazodone and trimipramine are the most used in this context. However, they are unpredictable and unreliable and should be used only to treat the primary illness of depression. The older tricyclic compounds are dangerous in overdose. Antipsychotic drugs such as chlorpromazine can be quite sedative but the risk of side effects, particularly movement disorders, precludes their use except in psychotic patients.

Residual Effects

Ideally a hypnotic should be active only during the night but to be effective it should not only induce sleep quickly but maintain it for a prolonged period, which results in a risk of excessive residual sedation. Residual effects comprise both subjective feelings of sedation and objective impairment of psychomotor and cognitive functioning occurring during the day following night-time ingestion. Such effects are related to both the pharmacokinetics of the drug and the dose given. The first benzodiazepines marketed as hypnotics were relatively long-acting and in response to studies showing residual impairment, shorter acting compounds were synthesised but these have produced other residual problems.

Residual effects have most frequently been studied in normal volunteer subjects. All benzodiazepine hypnotics produce some decrement in performance the day after night-time ingestion. This decrement is strongly related to dose but not consistently to half-life, although longer acting compounds generally show more impairment. The type of performance that is impaired after a single dose of a hypnotic is similar to that after acute doses of anxiolytic benzodiazepines administered during the day, i.e. speed of performance, acquisition of new material and anterograde memory. Few studies have examined effects after repeated doses but it seems that some tolerance develops. Despite build-up of plasma levels of the hypnotic, no further deterioration has been found after consecutive nights of administration.

A few studies have attempted to examine residual effects in patients with sleep disorders. These patients do not differ from controls in the pattern of effects shown but the decrement is less profound and sometimes absent at equivalent dose levels. The elderly are more likely to suffer adverse reactions to benzodiazepine hypnotics because of altered pharmacokinetics especially in the distribution and elimination of certain agents. These drugs have been found to be frequently implicated in drug-associated hospital admissions in elderly patients and the incidence of adverse effects such as confusion and ataxia increases with age. Such effects are reflected in measures of performance and cognition which show decrements after lower doses in this population.

Shorter acting benzodiazepines were developed to act primarily on sleep-onset problems and to lessen residual effects. In single dose studies with normal subjects, there is often less residual impairment but this has not been confirmed after repeated doses or in insomniac patients. In fact the very short acting triazolam may produce early morning insomnia, daytime anxiety and memory impairment.

Newer hypnotics such as zopiclone and zolpidem do not seem to differ substantially from the benzodiazepines. Residual effects seem to be related to dose and are less profound in those suffering from sleep disorders.

Rebound and Withdrawal

It is now clearly established that when a short- or even medium-acting hypnotic drug is abruptly discontinued, the patient may complain of insomnia for a night or two, which is worse than that for which the hypnotic was originally prescribed. Sleep laboratory studies have confirmed these subjective complaints, latency to sleep onset and wakefulness during the night being particularly affected. The phenomenon is an example of receptor rebound and is found with almost all drugs which act on receptors including beta-adrenoceptor blocking agents and histamine antagonists.

Rebound insomnia is not always easily discernible. It is common after cessation of short- or medium-acting drugs but uncommon after long-acting hypnotics are stopped. Even so, it is rarely present for more than one night. Consequently, night-by-night analyses of data are essential for its detection. Dosage is also critical. It is readily apparent after stopping triazolam in high dose (0.5 mg) but less apparent after treatment with 0.25 mg. Tapering of the dose attenuates the rebound. Thus, three nights of tapering dosage after three nights of triazolam 0.5 mg resulted in about half the disruption following six nights of 0.5 mg and then abrupt discontinuation. Discontinuation of placebo itself was followed by some rebound indicating the importance of psychological factors.

Somewhat surprisingly, duration of use has little effect on the likelihood of rebound insomnia. However, individual factors are important, some subjects showing rebound quite consistently, others withdrawing from hypnotic medication with impunity. Subjects with rebound insomnia tend to be poor sleepers anyway, and to show greater drug effects than subjects not developing rebound insomnia.

The importance of rebound insomnia relates to whether it renders the patient more likely to revert to hypnotic medication with the danger of long-term use with dependence. Because clinical experience suggests that rebound insomnia may pose management problems, further studies both within and outside sleep laboratories are needed.

The relationship of rebound insomnia to true withdrawal syndromes is unclear. A withdrawal syndrome is generally defined as including newly-emergent symptoms, i.e. symptoms which develop on withdrawal not previously experienced by the patient. Withdrawal phenomena can develop on stopping an hypnotic benzodiazepine after long-term use. The clinical picture and general management are identical to those related to the withdrawal of benzodiazepine anxiolytics (see p. 97).

In the UK, the main abuse problem with the benzodiazepines concerns the intravenous use of temazepam. This topic is dealt with in the chapter on anxiolytics (see p. 99).

NARCOLEPSY AND THE HYPERSOMNIAS

Hypersomnia means too much sleep and usually implies excessive sleeping or drowsiness during the day. It may present as a feature of atypical depression. Sleep laboratory and more recently 24-hour ambulatory monitoring has helped establish the abnormal sleep patterns in these conditions. The best-studied is narcolepsy.

Narcolepsy comprises persistently falling asleep under unusual circumstances. This is coupled with one of two other features, cataplexy or frequent sleep paralysis. The sleep attacks comprise irresistible urges to sleep during the daytime often at inappropriate or even dangerous times such as driving. The sufferer sleeps for a few minutes up to half an hour and awakes feeling refreshed. Cataplexy consists of abrupt attacks of profound muscle weakness which may result in the patient dropping helpless to the ground. Laughter or anger may trigger an attack. Sleep paralysis is a terrifying state in which the subject lies awake but cannot move without an extreme effort of will. There is a dissociation of sleep and dream that occur in REM sleep from the mechanisms of motor control.

The prevalence of narcolepsy is unclear but an informed guess is of 20 000 sufferers in the UK. Intriguingly, there is a strong relationship between narcolepsy and a particular immunological subtype (HLA DR2). The condition is strongly genetically determined.

The established treatment is with dexamphetamine, methylphenidate or mazindol. This usually controls the daytime sleepiness. However, they are attended by the usual problems of tolerance, dependence and rebound hypersomnia. The minimal effective dose must be attained and intermittent treatment may be necessary to combat the tolerance. The cataplexy is satisfactorily controlled by clomipramine, the tricyclic antidepressant, which might be construed as evidence that 5-HT mechanisms are involved. MAO inhibitors can also be effective but must never be given in combination with clomipramine.

Other causes of hypersomnia include lesions of the hypothalamus such as tumours and cysts. In 'sleeping sickness' (trypanosomiasis), parasites infest that area of the brain. Encephalitis may be associated with inversion of the sleep rhythm and with hypersomnia.

COMBINED TREATMENTS

Both pharmacological and non-pharmacological therapies have been shown to be effective in the treatment of sleep disorders. Unfortunately there is a lack of systematic research comparing and combining the two approaches. One study has compared relaxation plus stimulus control with triazolam 0.5 mg for four weeks. Triazolam had an immediate effect on sleep onset and total sleep time but this declined at follow-up whereas behavioural treatment had a slow, sustained effect which started after the second week's treatment, became equivalent to the drug after four weeks and was superior at follow-up (five weeks later). There is a need for further evaluations.

SUMMARY

Problems with sleep and hypnotic use are common. Insomnia is a subjective complaint and varies considerably between individuals. There are many causes for poor sleep. Taking a careful history of the condition and educating the patient about good sleep hygiene are the first line of treatment. Patients who are unresponsive to these measures may need more structured psychological therapy or short-term or intermittent drug treatment. Hypnotic drugs can cause residual impairment especially in the elderly. Rebound insomnia may occur after cessation of short- or medium-acting drugs. Narcolepsy is a rare condition.

FURTHER READING

Benca, R.M., Obermeyer, W.H., Thisted, R.A. et al. (1992) Sleep and psychiatric disorders. *Archives of General Psychiatry* **49**, 651–668.
Bond, A. and Lader, M. (1981) After effects of sleeping drugs. In *Psychopharmacology of Sleep* (Wheatley, D., ed.). Raven Press, New York, pp. 177–197.
Espie, C.A. (1991) *The Psychological Treatment of Insomnia*. Wiley, Chichester.
Goa, K.L. and Heel, R.C. (1986) Zopiclone. A review of its pharmacodynamic and pharmacokinetic properties and therapeutic efficacy as an hypnotic. *Drugs* **32**, 48–65.
Greenblatt, D.J., Miller, L.G. and Shader, R.I. (1990) Neurochemical and pharmacokinetic correlates of the clinical action of benzodiazepine hypnotic drugs. *American Journal of Medicine* **88** (suppl. 3A), 18S–24S.
Hauri, P. (1982) *The Sleep Disorders*. Upjohn, Kalamazoo, MI.
Johnson, L.C. and Chernik, D.A. (1982) Sedative-hypnotics and human performance. *Psychopharmacology*. **76**, 101–113.

Kruse, W. H.-H. (1990) Problems and pitfalls in the use of benzodiazepines in the elderly. *Drug Safety* **5**, 328–344.

Lacks, P. (1987) *Behavioral Treatment for Persistent Insomnia.* Pergamon Press, New York.

Lader, M. (1992) The Medical Management of Insomnia in General Practice. *Round Table Series* No. 28, Royal Society of Medicine, London.

Lader, M. and Lawson, C. (1987) Sleep studies and rebound insomnia: methodological problems, laboratory findings, and clinical implications. *Clinical Neuropharmacology* **10**, 291–312.

Langtry, H.D. and Benfield, P. (1990) Zolpidem. A review of its pharmacodynamic and pharmacokinetic properties and therapeutic potential. *Drugs* **40**, 291–313.

Maczaj, M. (1993) Pharmacological treatment of insomnia. *Drugs* **45**, 44–55.

McClusky, H.Y., Milby, J.B., Switzer, P.K. et al. (1991) Efficacy of behavioral versus triazolam treatment in persistent sleep-onset insomnia. *American Journal of Psychiatry* **148**, 121–126.

Morgan, K., Dallosso, H., Ebrahim, S. et al. (1988) Prevalence, frequency, and duration of hypnotic drug use among the elderly living at home. *British Medical Journal* **296**, 601–602.

Morin, C.M., Culbert, J.P. and Schwartz, S.M. (1994) Nonpharmacological interventions for insomnia: a meta-analysis of treatment efficacy. *American Journal of Psychiatry* **151**, 1172–1180.

Roehrs, T., Merlotti, L., Zorick, F. et al. (1992) Rebound insomnia in normals and patients with insomnia after abrupt and tapered discontinuation. *Psychopharmacology* **108**, 67–71.

Tyrer, P. (1993) Withdrawal from hypnotic drugs. *British Medical Journal* **306**, 706–708.

Woods, J.H., Katz, J.L. and Winger, G. (1987) Abuse liability of benzodiazepines. *Pharmacological Reviews* **39**, 251–413.

Chapter 9

TREATMENT OF DEPRESSION

In this chapter, the treatment of depression is discussed. There are several types of antidepressant drug and the efficacy and profile of unwanted effects of each are described. The use of cognitive therapy and interpersonal therapy in the treatment of depression is reviewed as well as their combination with drug treatment.

Clinical depression can be described as a persistent lowering of mood or a pervasive loss of interest which has been present for at least two weeks and which represents a change from previous functioning. In its more severe forms, the low mood may be unremitting throughout the day or it may be worse in the morning with some improvement later in the day (diurnal variation). In milder forms, mood may be more reactive to minor life events. Although mood change is the prime feature of depression it is accompanied by a number of other features (Figure 9.1). There is a sense of loss which is reflected in loss of interest and pleasure and a difficulty in executing even simple tasks, leading to low activity levels. Somatic symptoms abound. Sleep and appetite are often affected. Usually this is seen as a lowering of function but occasionally oversleeping and overeating are seen. Fatigue is common and there may be numerous other physical complaints. Sometimes overt psychomotor symptoms are apparent either in the form of an inability to keep still (agitation) or in a slowness to start or complete a movement or train of thought (retardation). There may be other mood changes: anxiety is often increased sometimes to a level of panic so that it is difficult to determine which is the primary complaint, and irritability may also be present. Cognitive symptoms include changes in the way in which depressed people think about themselves, their world and their future. Feelings of inadequacy lead to low self-esteem and a feeling of hopelessness is linked to the risk of suicide.

Depression can be classified according to severity. In the most severe form, negative beliefs may become delusional or psychotic. Depression usually occurs in episodes with natural remission in between. A single episode of depression is often related to stressful events or situations (Figure 9.2). These may be major or minor life events associated with loss such as bereavement, physical illnesses, changes at work or relationship problems. Sometimes

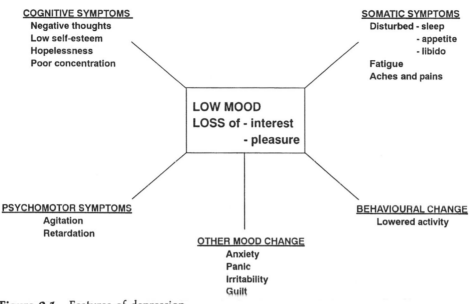

Figure 9.1   Features of depression

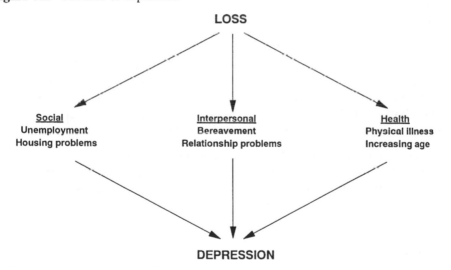

Figure 9.2   Precipitants of depression

events which seem advantageous or positive, such as promotion or childbirth, also precipitate depression because the individual doubts his/her ability to cope with this change. When two or more episodes of depression are experienced, it is described as recurrent. When episodes of depression alternate with episodes of mania or elevated mood the disorder is described as bipolar or manic-depressive psychosis (Chapter 10). A less severe chronic lowering of mood may be termed 'dysthymia'.

BIOLOGICAL HYPOTHESES OF DEPRESSION

One of the earliest observations was that reserpine, an antipsychotic drug introduced from Indian herbal medicine, depleted nerve endings of monoamines and could precipitate retardation and depression. It was postulated that depression was related to a deficit of monoamines in the brain, mania to a surfeit. The finding that both tricyclic antidepressants and monoamine oxidase antidepressants increased the availability of brain amines supported this notion. The problem, however, was to demonstrate these abnormalities in depressed patients. Technical difficulties hamper the study of the intact human although these may be partly circumvented using modern neuroimaging techniques.

Some postmortem studies have relied on the knowledge that many, but definitely not all, people who deliberately commit suicide are clinically depressed at the time. Many factors have to be considered such as mode of death, previous drug history, current therapy and time between death and estimation of brain amines. Detailed neuropathological examinations are necessary to exclude possible degenerative disorders. Some evidence suggests that postsynaptic 5-HT$_2$ receptors are increased in the cerebral cortex of depressives. Other serotonin receptors appear normal. Perhaps the most robust finding is that a subgroup of depressed patients with low concentrations of the serotonin metabolite, 5-HIAA, in the cerebrospinal fluid are more likely to show violent suicidal behaviour.

Another popular approach is the neuroendocrine one. This exploits a range of probe drugs which release various hormones, mostly from the pituitary. The cortisol system has received much attention. Thus, some depressives show decreased sensitivity to the suppression of cortisol secretion by the drug, dexamethasone. This test, the dexamethasone suppression test, (DST) was exhaustively evaluated around 10 years ago but was found to be too nonspecific. Another system studied was the thyroid: some depressives show decreased sensitivity to the release of thyroid stimulating hormone (TSH) by thyrotropin releasing hormone (TRH). Finally, growth hormone release to the adrenergic agonist clonidine is blunted in depressives. Overall, neuroendocrine abnormalities are fairly well established as a feature of depression but both their pathogenesis and interpretation remain poorly understood.

Because brain receptor function is difficult to study in humans, either with neuroimaging, postmortem or neuroendocrine techniques, 'models' have been set up using circulating blood platelets or lymphocytes. This presupposes that receptor abnormalities occur throughout the body. The serotonin uptake site on the platelet has been found to be reduced significantly in depressed patients but other receptors seem less consistently altered.

Another approach has been to attempt to manipulate neurotransmitter function by interfering with synthesis, release and inactivation. Some of these manoeuvres are essentially therapeutic in nature, for example, the use of L-tryptophan to increase brain serotonin and thereby act as an adjunct to antidepressive treatment. The opposite has also been attempted. As amino acids compete for uptake into the brain, administration of a drink containing the amino acids that compete with tryptophan results in a marked but transient decrease in brain serotonin. Drug-free depressives show no immediate mood changes but about a third have a transient elevation of mood when the normal tryptophan-containing diet is re-instituted. Depressives in clinical remission after six to eight weeks of SSRI treatment experience a transient relapse during acute tryptophan depletion.

In conclusion, many lines of evidence point to the involvement of brain amines in the depressive process. Of these amines, the evidence is strongest for a malfunctioning of serotonin. It is unclear whether the changes described are primary or secondary to some other abnormality. Nor is it clear what biochemical factors are involved in the pathogenesis of these abnormalities. The possibility of genetically determined predispositions is being studied, so far with tantalising possibilities but no consistent evidence.

ANTIDEPRESSANT DRUGS

In the 1950s, two groups of antidepressant drugs were discovered, the tricyclic antidepressants (TCAs) named after their chemical structure, and the monoamine oxidase inhibitors (MAOIs) referring to their main biochemical actions. A great deal of heated debate attended the use of the MAOIs as their adverse and even dangerous side-effects became quickly apparent.

It must be remembered that neuropharmacology was still in its infancy, only a few neurotransmitters identified, and receptor pharmacology almost unknown. It was quickly apparent that the mode of action of antidepressants must be quite complex, one compelling piece of evidence being the delay in onset of the clinical antidepressant effect in contrast to the rapid effect of antidepressants on brain amines in animals. Nevertheless, many compounds were screened for the ability to alter amine disposition in the brains of animals in the short-term. Only when it became apparent that some compounds found effective in the clinic had anomalous effects on amines did the search for newer and better antidepressants widen.

Very many TCAs were introduced, most of which are closely akin in pharmacological and clinical properties to imipramine and amitriptyline, the first two of this class. Later, compounds with some benefits were developed, for example, lofepramine with its lower incidence of autonomic side-effects, and amoxapine with a more rapid onset of action. More selective TCAs were sought: the older compounds affected both serotonin and noradrenaline and it was thought that compounds affecting one or other selectively might be particularly effective in specific but so far undefined and undetectable groups of patients. The newer compounds were selective either on noradrenaline (e.g. maprotiline) or serotonin. A whole group of compounds of the latter type has been developed — the selective serotonin re-uptake inhibitors (SSRIs).

Meanwhile, attempts were being made to lessen the toxicity and adverse effects of the MAOIs. The older compounds blocked all forms of MAO indiscriminately and irreversibly. A selective MAO-B inhibitor, selegeline, was found to be a poor antidepressant but useful in Parkinson's Disease. Then, reversible inhibitors of monoamine oxidase A (RIMAs) were developed, of which one, moclobemide, has been marketed. Many other compounds are in development and the range of pharmacological profiles is now very wide. Despite this variety, the efficacies are all equivalent although the side-effect profiles differ markedly.

TRICYCLIC ANTIDEPRESSANTS

Imipramine was the first of these compounds to be introduced. In an early account (Kuhn, 1958) of his open clinical observations of imipramine in depressed patients, Roland Kuhn described the dosage regimens required, the failure of some patients to respond, the characteristics of those who did, the delay in onset of action, and the numerous unwanted effects. Imipramine was introduced into clinical practice in a rather muted way but its usage soon became routine. Other tricyclic compounds were synthesised, evaluated and marketed. TCAs have also been used in other indications such as nocturnal enuresis and chronic pain.

Imipramine

Imipramine is rapidly absorbed, being detected in the plasma after a few minutes after absorption on an empty stomach. Distribution is rapid and imipramine readily crosses into the brain. It is extensively metabolised in the liver and has many metabolites. The most important is desipramine. Together, imipramine and desipramine have an effective half-life in the plasma of about 24 hours, so it takes four to five days for steady-state levels to be attained.

Wide variations in plasma concentrations are found in patients. The ratio of imipramine to desipramine is about unity but also varies from subject to subject.

Pharmacology

Several neurotransmitter systems are altered by the administration of imipramine, among them being serotonin, noradrenaline and acetylcholine. Imipramine blocks the active transport systems for noradrenaline and serotonin which take the released transmitter out of the synaptic cleft back into the presynaptic neuron. Imipramine is more potent in inhibiting the uptake of serotonin than of noradrenaline, desipramine the reverse. Dopamine is affected only weakly. Adaptive changes occur within the neuron and in receptors to overcome the uptake blockade. The synthesis of the above neurotransmitters is reduced, as is turnover. The effects on brain amines are therefore quite complex. Receptors also alter and with a time-course closer to that of clinical response than are the amine changes. In particular $5\text{-}HT_2$ receptors diminish in number ('down-regulate').

Imipramine interacts with several other types of drug. It can prevent and partly reverse the depressant effects of amine-depleting drugs such as reserpine and tetrabenazine. Conversely, it potentiates amphetamines and other central stimulants. It prevents the uptake into nerve endings of tyramine and some obsolescent anti-hypertensive drugs such as guanethidine.

Other TCAs

Amitriptyline is similar to imipramine in its pharmacology and clinical effects although it is more sedative and has more noticeable anticholinergic effects. It is metabolised in a similar way (by demethylation to nortriptyline) and also has a fairly long plasma half-life. It has been evaluated in many clinical trials and again like imipramine, is often used as a standard comparator in the evaluation of new antidepressants. Amitriptyline is one of the more dangerous TCAs in overdose.

Nortriptyline is the main metabolite of amitriptyline but is available as a TCA in its own right. Its pharmacokinetics have been extensively studied because it was the first compound for which sensitive and accurate methods of measurement were developed. Treatment with standard dosage results in up to 30-fold variation in steady-state concentrations. Genetic factors strongly influence metabolism. Clinically, nortriptyline is as effective as other TCAs but is less sedative and rather less useful in agitated and anxious patients.

Desipramine is similar to imipramine but is less sedative. *Trimipramine* is more sedative and is particularly useful in the depressed insomniac. *Butriptyline* has the same side-chain as trimipramine and is also sedative whereas *protriptyline* is quite stimulant and may induce restlessness and insomnia.

Dothiepin is the most widely used TCA in the UK and resembles amitriptyline in many of its properties including sedation, anticholinergic effects and toxicity in overdose. *Doxepin* is less sedative. *Amoxapine* has a fairly rapid onset of action but may induce extrapyramidal side-effects on occasion.

Maprotiline is chemically a tricyclic drug with a linked structure in the molecule. It closely resembles other TCAs but selectively blocks the re-uptake of noradrenaline. It lowers the convulsive threshold more than other TCAs and is therefore more likely to induce fits.

Clomipramine is an interesting TCA. It was first marketed in Europe about 20 years ago but much more recently in the USA. It is a powerful and selective 5-HT re-uptake inhibitor, although its main metabolite chlordesipramine preferentially inhibits noradrenaline re-uptake. It has become widely used to treat depression and is favoured as a treatment in otherwise refractory depression. It is used also to treat obsessive-compulsive disorders and panic disorders (see Chapter 7). Its adverse effects are usually mild to moderate and well-tolerated and stem mainly from its anticholinergic properties.

Lofepramine is also unusual. It is a TCA, structurally resembling imipramine but with a much bulkier side-chain. It is, however, largely metabolised to desipramine. The side-chain seems to interfere with binding to acetylcholine receptors so the side-effect profile of lofepramine is superior to that of other TCAs, although some incidence of dry mouth is reported. It is particularly well-tolerated by the elderly. Its efficacy is indistinguishable from other TCAs. Somewhat unexpectedly, it is much safer in overdose than other TCAs and adverse effects on cardiac function are minimal.

Clinical Uses

The main indication for the TCAs is major depressive disorder. However, other forms of depression such as dysthymic disorder, depression in early dementia, depression in schizophrenic patients and depressive reactions in the context of personality disorders respond to a TCA to some extent. It is generally believed that the more 'biological' the depression, i.e. with features such as insomnia and anorexia, the more likely is response to occur: unfortunately, the evidence to support this clinical impression is weak.

Many trials now support the clinical efficacy of the TCAs as compared with placebo. Roughly speaking, about two-thirds of patients with major depressive disorder respond adequately to a TCA as compared with about a third to placebo. Nevertheless many such double-blind comparative trials fail to show a significant difference and the impression is that this proportion has gradually increased over the past two decades. Explanations for this include the non-specific therapeutic effect of frequent assessments and ratings, the recruitment of less ill patients or even depressed volunteers, and the lower tolerance of adverse effects by patients, investigators and ethical committees.

The symptoms which improve significantly with TCAs cover a wide spectrum from insomnia to feelings of guilt and worthlessness and lack of motivation. The core symptom of depressed mood, sadness, etc. shows a clear response. The time course of response is still a matter of some controversy. The general view is that there is a delay in onset of action of two to three weeks, or even more. Detailed evaluations have suggested that improvement in somatic symptoms occurs earlier, and is usually the first feature to be noted. Patients remark that they sleep more deeply and longer and wake feeling more refreshed and better able to face the ensuing day. General activation also improves, the patient becoming more alert, able to attend and concentrate, and retardation lessens. Eventually, the depressive mood starts to lift: it is this element of the illness which may be delayed for two to four weeks from the initiation of TCA therapy and may give the superficial impression of overall delay. In anxious or phobic depressives, the anxiety may be slow to respond or selectively refractory to treatment.

Factors associated with a favourable response to a TCA have been shown in a series of controlled studies to include few previous episodes, insidious onset, brief duration of illness and lack of precipitating causes. Patients with anorexia, weight loss, early wakening, and psychomotor slowing usually respond most adequately whereas deluded patients may do badly and often need the addition of an antipsychotic drug. In schizophrenic patients, a TCA may increase hostility and agitation, and activate delusions and thought disorder. Its effect on depressive symptoms may be disappointing. Despite this, and because of the frequency of depression in such patients, many schizophrenics are treated with an antipsychotic and a TCA. However, fixed combinations of this type have little to commend them.

Unwanted Effects

The unwanted side-effects of the TCA (Table 9.1) are usually minor, transient and not troublesome but with some patients they are so marked that they lessen compliance or may result in total failure to take the medication. The assessment of these unwanted effects is complicated by some of them, e.g. constipation and dry mouth, being somatic symptoms of depression itself. It

Table 9.1   Common side-effects of antidepressants

Antidepressant	Side-effect
TCAs	Anticholinergic: dry mouth constipation tremor Sedation
Newer type	Some sedation, nausea
SSRIs	Gastrointestinal: nausea loss of appetite Some insomnia Initial increase in anxiety
MAOIs	Postural hypotension Autonomic Interaction with tyramine
RIMAs	Some nausea, insomnia

is often difficult to disentangle the two. A clue may be given by the time-relationships as drug-related effects typically occur one to three hours after taking the TCA.

CNS Effects

A common side-effect of many TCAs is drowsiness and torpor. It is an unpleasant, heavy feeling akin to that of the sedative antihistamines. As well as drowsiness, the patient may feel light-headed and detached from reality. The sedation comes on quickly in the first few days and then lessens over the next week or so although it may not totally disappear. Thinking, attention, concentration and especially memory can be demonstrably impaired (see below).

A persistent fine tremor may be induced, especially in the elderly. Some TCAs such as amoxapine and amitriptyline may occasionally cause extrapyramidal reactions. Rare neurotoxic reactions have been reported with ataxia, nystagmus, dysarthria and tremor.

The convulsive threshold is lowered by most TCAs, maprotiline being most likely to do this at clinical dosage. As with all antidepressant therapy, a hypomanic reaction may be induced, bipolar patients being most at risk.

The anticholinergic effects may be associated with confusional reactions, especially in the elderly. Visual illusions are early symptoms and may progress to unformed visual hallucinations. This type of reaction is most likely when a TCA is combined with an anticholinergic antipsychotic drug. The abrupt withdrawal of a TCA may be followed by an akathisia-like syndrome with restlessness, anxiety, malaise, muscular aching, nausea, vomiting and dizziness.

Cardiovascular System

Postural hypotension is a common reaction to a TCA in the young, the old and the physically debilitated. The heart then speeds up to try and compensate for this. The hypotension usually wanes but may persist to some extent.

ECG changes are complex. TCAs prolong conduction mechanisms in the heart. Slowing or speeding up of the heart, irregularities and extra beats may supervene, especially on higher doses and routinely after suicidal overdoses. Suspicion has been aroused that these changes may cause sudden death but the evidence for this supposition is scanty. Lofepramine, some newer compounds and the SSRIs are much safer, even in overdose.

Gastrointestinal System

Anticholinergic effects include reduced bowel motility with constipation which can become quite severe or even culminate in paralysis of the ileum. Relaxation of the oesophagus may cause a hiatus hernia. Acid formation in the stomach is diminished by the TCAs which may therefore be appropriate in depressed patients with peptic ulcer.

Genitourinary System

Many TCAs are powerfully anticholinergic and thereby increase the tone of the bladder sphincter. This results in difficulty in urination but this is usually only of clinical significance in patients with pre-existing pathology like prostatic enlargement. Elderly males should be asked about their bladder function before being given a TCA.

Delayed ejaculation and orgasm is another common side-effect. Erectile dysfunction and loss of libido may also occur. Often the patient already has sexual dysfunction related to his depressive illness and may only notice drug-related problems after some weeks of treatment.

Metabolic and Endocrine

Patients on TCAs often report a craving for carbohydrates. This can result in a substantial increase in weight, and compliance may be affected.

Endocrine effects involve the pituitary-gonad axis and include menstrual irregularities, breast enlargement and secretion of milk in women, impotence, breast and testicular swelling in men.

Other Effects

Pupillary dilatation and loss of accommodation with blurring of vision can prove troublesome. Intraocular pressure tends to rise so TCAs must be avoided in patients with glaucoma. Increase in sweating has been described, a paradoxical effect.

Minor side-effects include headache, fatigue, nausea, anorexia, soreness of the mouth, peculiar taste sensations and nightmares. Liver function tests may be mildly impaired but occasionally jaundice may supervene. Allergic reactions include rashes and hives. Very occasionally, blood dyscrasias have been reported.

TCAs should be avoided in pregnancy wherever possible although no direct teratogenic link has ever been demonstrated. They should also be withheld from lactating mothers.

Interactions with Other Drugs

The sedative actions of TCAs are potentiated by and in turn potentiate the sedative actions of many psychotropic drugs such as alcohol, the hypnotic/sedatives, antipsychotics and the older antihistamines. Patients taking TCAs must be warned about drowsiness, urged not to drive and adjured to avoid alcohol.

Stimulant effects of amphetamine are increased, as are those of some other sympathomimetics. Potentiation of phenothiazines is a problem at high dose and may result in confusion, constipation, dry mouth and urinary retention.

Interactions with cardiovascular drugs are complex depending on the mechanism of action of the drug. Expert review of medication may be necessary when treating a depressed, hypertensive patient.

Overdose

Overdose is a major problem with the TCAs because they are toxic in overdose and are prescribed for depressed patients who often have suicidal ideas or intentions. The standard TCAs such as imipramine and amitriptyline can induce toxic effects at doses over about 600 mg, i.e. four times the usual therapeutic dose. Doses over 2.5 g are likely to prove lethal. Symptoms usually appear within four hours and commonly include dry mouth, blurred vision, dilated pupils, rapid pulse, extrapyramidal signs such as rigidity and either drowsiness or excitement. The cardiovascular effects of overdosage are the most life-threatening, the arrhythmias in particular. All types of heart conduction defects can occur and may culminate in ventricular tachycardia, fibrillation and death. Myocardial depression also occurs. Respiration is depressed and this results in lack of oxygen to the heart and further toxicity. Central effects comprise excitement or coma with shock. Convulsions may occur especially in children. Other effects include increased reflexes, muscle twitching and paralysis of the bowel and bladder.

Care in prescribing can minimise the risk of overdose. Identification of the potential suicidal patient is a preliminary to the choice of medication. A person who has attempted suicide before or a recently widowed elderly man are examples of patients at risk. Newer compounds like the SSRIs, lofepramine, mianserin, etc. should be seriously considered. Prescriptions of TCAs should be for conservative amounts but even a week's supply at full dosage can prove lethal. Entrusting the medication to a responsible relative or friend is a wise precaution. The problem of accidental overdosage among children is a worrying one but childproof containers may also prove very difficult for the elderly arthritic to open.

NEWER TRICYCLIC-TYPE COMPOUNDS

A few compounds have been introduced as antidepressant which resemble some but not all aspects of the TCAs. They are sometimes called 'atypical' compounds or more pretentiously, 'Second-Generation Antidepressants'.

Mianserin is a true tetracyclic chemically and has some unusual pharmacological properties. It impairs noradrenaline and serotonin uptake only weakly, but also blocks presynaptic noradrenergic synapses thereby increasing noradrenaline turnover in the brain like some other antidepressants. In humans it is devoid of significant anticholinergic actions but it is rather sedative. It has little effect on the heart and is safe in overdose. It has some propensity to induce agranulocytosis (drop in white blood cells) particularly in the elderly.

Trazodone is chemically unrelated to other antidepressants and acts mainly on serotonin mechanisms. Its efficacy is similar to standard TCAs but it is quite sedative and has been used extensively to treat depressed patients with insomnia. It has few anticholinergic side-effects and has low cardiotoxicity and toxicity in overdose. It is well-tolerated by the elderly. A rare side-effect is persistent and painful penile erection.

Nefazodone is a recently introduced drug which both blocks serotonin re-uptake and $5-HT_2$ receptors. This seems to confer a favourable side-effect profile but experience with the compound is very limited as yet.

Buproprion is available in the USA but not in the UK. It has some stimulant effects. *Viloxazine* is chemically different from the TCAs, and blocks noradrenaline re-uptake. Although not regarded as particularly efficacious, it has few side-effects apart from some nausea and vomiting.

Venlafaxine is a novel antidepressant which has powerful effects in blocking the re-uptake of both noradrenaline and serotonin, but lacks effects on cholinergic, histaminergic or adrenergic receptors. It has antidepressant properties equivalent to TCAs but with a superior side-effect profile. It may have a somewhat more rapid onset of action.

SELECTIVE SEROTONIN RE-UPTAKE INHIBITORS (SSRIs)

It was believed that concentrating on one neurotransmitter might expedite the development of drugs with enhanced efficacy, at least in a subgroup of depressed patients. Thus, it was postulated that a proportion (unspecified) of depressed patients had associated impairment of serotonin- rather than noradrenaline-related function and that administering a drug selective for serotonin would be a more focused approach than a non-specific TCA. It was known that clomipramine was a potent and selective serotonin uptake inhibitor but was metabolised in the body to a metabolite more selective on noradrenaline re-uptake, the practical upshot being loss of selectivity. The first selective compound to be developed was zimeldine, and this too lost some selectivity on metabolism. However, it proved to be neurotoxic and was withdrawn. Another, indalpine, also had adverse effects and was only available in France.

Fluvoxamine was the first SSRI to be marketed in Europe which is still available. It was not introduced to the USA where fluoxetine was the first and quickly became very widely prescribed. Sertraline followed and then paroxetine. Others such as citalopram are available in some countries. These compounds differ with respect to pharmacokinetics and to side-effect profile. They have excited a great deal of interest and controversy, not least because they are much more expensive than the older TCAs.

Efficacy

As to be expected with recently-developed drugs, a range of controlled trials — some with placebo, some active comparator, and many with both — attest to the efficacy of the SSRIs. The studies usually involve patients with major depressive disorder of moderate severity. Both fixed and flexible doses have been used. Meta-analyses of these studies have shown that the SSRIs are consistently superior to placebo but are no more effective than the standard TCAs. Nor is there any evidence of differential responsiveness among subgroups of patients. Some differences in response patterns may occur. Thus, the SSRIs are non-sedative or even somewhat stimulant, so insomnia is slower to respond than to a TCA. Anxiety levels may increase over the first few days but then an anxiolytic effect is often more apparent than with a TCA. The time-course of response for an SSRI is similar to that for a TCA.

SSRIs have been used in panic disorder and obsessive-compulsive disorder (see Chapter 7). Other indications that have been explored include substance abuse disorders, aggressive behaviour, and eating disorders such as bulimia. The rationale is generally that as serotonin is involved in some way in all of these disorders, altering its disposition with an SSRI might prove beneficial.

Unwanted Effects

Although the overall efficacy of the SSRIs does not differ materially from that of the TCAs, the side-effect and toxicity profiles diverge substantially (Table 9.1), usually to the advantage of the SSRIs. One crude measure of how well a drug is tolerated is to count the number of patients who drop out of controlled clinical trials because of adverse effects. In general, this figure is lower for the SSRI than the comparator TCA. Obviously, flexible dosage schedules should be better tolerated than fixed dosages and this must be taken into account.

Many of the SSRI side-effects are closely dose-related so that establishing the optimal dose for the best risk/benefit ratio is important. The early development of fluoxetine was pitched at too high a dose level (up to 80 mg/day) resulting in unacceptable toxicity. This largely vanished at 20 mg/day.

The commonest side-effects with an SSRI are gastrointestinal in nature. Nausea is usually transient and dose-related but can persist and result in drop-out or poor compliance. Loss of appetite is more pronounced in overweight patients and fluoxetine found an early, wide and strictly-speaking non-licensed indication as a dieting pill. Diarrhoea is usually not persistent. CNS effects are quite common but usually minor in nature. Increased anxiety and nervousness occurs, as noted earlier, and insomnia may be intensified. Tremor may occasionally occur and some extrapyramidal reactions such as dyskinesia have been documented.

Claims were made that fluoxetine was occasionally associated with the onset of intense, intrusive and violent suicidal ideation and preoccupation. Violent crimes in the USA committed by fluoxetine users were sometimes ascribed to the drug — the so-called 'Prozac defense'. Such effects were rarely seen in Europe, or at least were not reported. After intensive discussion and debate, heated but not enlightened, the controversy dampened down. If such reactions do occur, they are very uncommon, and have been recorded with some TCAs as well. Any depressed patient, whatever the treatment, needs careful supervision with particular attention paid to suicidal risk.

SSRI side-effects are anorgasmia and delayed ejaculation. Dry mouth and blurred vision are also reported. On the positive side, cardiovascular effects are minimal and all the SSRIs seem safer in overdose than TCAs.

The combination of an SSRI and an MAOI is potentially very hazardous, resulting in the 'serotonin syndrome'. They should never be combined and because fluoxetine and its metabolite norfluoxetine are very long-acting compounds, several weeks must elapse between stopping fluoxetine and starting an MAOI, even moclobemide.

The debate continues as to whether the better tolerability and safety of the SSRIs justifies the price differential over the very cheap TCAs. The wisest course is to make a decision appropriate to each patient taking into account age, previous drug history, need to maintain alertness, etc.

MONOAMINE OXIDASE INHIBITORS (MAOIs)

These compounds are much less used than the TCAs, the SSRIs, and related compounds. However, they have a complex pharmacology and the introduction of a selective MAOI, moclobemide, has revived interest in the group. As with the TCAs, the relationship of MAO inhibition to clinical response is still not clear. Isoniazid, and a closely-related compound iproniazid, were introduced in the late 1950s to treat tuberculosis. Both, particularly the latter, were noted to induce overactivity and euphoria. About this time the effects of iproniazid in inhibiting MAO were noted, leading to the hypothesis that stimulation and mood elevation was related to an increase in brain amines. Many depressed patients were treated with iproniazid. Unfortunately the drug produced an unacceptably high incidence of jaundice and liver damage. New MAOIs were developed and introduced but most were still somewhat toxic. Interactions with certain foodstuffs and with other drugs such as sympatho-mimetic amines became apparent and further reduced the popularity of these compounds. Of the older MAOIs, phenelzine and tranylcypromine retained some adherents who prescribed them in special situations.

Pharmacokinetics

All the first-generation MAOIs were irreversible inhibitors of MAO. Consequently, once an adequate concentration in the body had been attained to effect this, the MAO remained inactive. When the MAOI was removed, up to two weeks could elapse before new enzyme was synthesised and brain amines were metabolised normally again.

Pharmacology

MAO is an enzyme which is widely distributed in the body. It is localised within the cell where its main function is to inactivate amines including noradrenaline, dopamine and serotonin. The activity of MAO is influenced by many factors including age, hormonal state and some bodily rhythms. MAO exists in two major forms (isoenzymes): MAO-A which breaks down noradrenaline and serotonin; MAO-B has little affinity for these compounds; both metabolise tyramine and dopamine. MAOI-selective drugs have been developed. Selegeline is a selective MAO-B inhibitor and is widely used to treat Parkinsonism; it has little antidepressant activity except at high doses when the selectivity is lessened.

The inhibition of MAO leads to the widespread accumulation of amines. Since an excess of MAO exists in cells, high levels of inhibition may be necessary before amines start to accumulate.

A single dose of an MAOI produces little detectable effect behaviourally or physiologically. Tranylcypromine in a large single dose can act as a stimulant. Like amphetamine, tranylcypromine releases noradrenaline from nerve endings and can block its re-uptake as well as its metabolism.

Clinical Uses

Early studies were large-scale but uncontrolled, and inevitably generated uncritical acclaim. Controlled trials were less impressive, especially in depressed inpatients. Nevertheless, the bulk of evidence suggests useful efficacy for phenelzine and tranylcypromine although the trend is for these drugs to be inferior to standard TCAs. Some trials have suggested that larger than usual doses of an MAOI are associated with better clinical responses than with standard recommended doses. For example, doses of 90 mg of phenelzine are often used when lower doses (45–75 mg/day) have failed to effect a worthwhile improvement. Treatment response may be delayed even longer than with a TCA — up to six weeks or more. Accordingly, a fair trial of treatment implies a high dose for several weeks.

Although overall MAOIs seem somewhat less effective than standard TCAs, claims have long been made that a particular subgroup of patients is especially responsive to the MAOIs. This subgroup is generally designated as suffering from 'atypical depression'. Although this term is often poorly defined, symptoms such as irritability, somatic anxiety, hypochondriasis and phobias are prominent in such patients. Controlled studies have only shown one consistent factor predicting response, namely, the presence of phobic anxiety.

Unwanted Effects

The most common and troublesome side-effect is postural hypotension (Table 9.1). Tolerance does not develop and the drop in blood pressure may cause dangerous faintness and may act as the limiting factor in increasing the dose. An unusual adverse effect is oedema (fluid swelling) in the legs or hands, often quite gross and sometimes unilateral. Restlessness and hyperactivity are particularly seen with tranylcypromine; patients with retardation may become agitated; schizophrenic patients may develop activation of their psychotic features; bipolar patients may be precipitated into mania. Rare effects include pins and needles in the fingers and toes, peripheral neuropathy and muscle twitches. The earlier drugs such as iproniazid, isocarboxazid and nialamide were associated with a jaundice caused by destruction of liver cells, which could be fatal.

Autonomic side-effects include dry mouth and skin, hesitancy of urination, blurring of vision and constipation. Changes in libido and delayed ejaculation may occur. Allergic skin reactions and drops in blood cell count have been recorded.

Drug and Dietary Interactions

Tyramine is produced by the breakdown of the amino acid tyrosine, a natural component of tissues. When tyramine is ingested it is usually inactivated by MAO. MAO inhibition prevents the breakdown of amines, both endogenous and dietary, in the gut wall and the liver. It also increases the noradrenaline stores throughout the body. Thus, tyramine reaches the general circulation and then blood vessels where it releases noradrenaline. This causes severe headache and a marked rise in blood pressure which can cause bleeding in the brain blood vessels and hence death. The list of foods which contain large amounts of tyramine (and some other amines) is fairly short. The main ones are some cheeses, meat and malt extracts and runner bean pods. Home-made beer, pickled herring, even caviare have been implicated. The food interactions are unpredictable and some patients break the rules without dire consequences.

More dangerous and predictable interactions occur with drugs. Amine drugs which release noradrenaline can cause hypertension. These include phenylephrine and phenylpropanolamine. Such drugs are available without prescription and are sold as nasal decongestants. Patients taking the older MAOIs are usually issued with a warning card by the dispensing pharmacist to carry with them. Other drugs which are potentiated are levodopa, used in the treatment of parkinsonism, and amphetamines.

Drugs acting on the serotonin system can be potentiated producing the serotonin syndrome characterised by restlessness, excitement, sweating, high temperature, muscular rigidity or twitching and pupillary dilatation. Coma and death may supervene. The drugs involved include TCAs acting powerfully on serotonin re-uptake such as clomipramine, and the SSRIs. Although a few psychiatrists do combine a TCA and an MAOI, they are very judicious in their choice, usually favouring trimipramine and phenelzine.

MAOIs also inhibit other enzymes and may interfere with the metabolism of a wide variety of drugs including pethidine and other opioids. Antihypertensive agents may also be potentiated.

Overdose

An overdose of an MAOI can be fatal. Signs are usually delayed for 12 hours or so and then headache, chest pain and restlessness progress to confusion and delirium. Attacks of high blood pressure may culminate in acute heart failure or intracranial haemorrhage. High body temperature and brisk reflexes are common.

REVERSIBLE INHIBITORS OF MONOAMINE OXIDASE (RIMAs)

Only one of these drugs, moclobemide is so far on the market, although a few others are in development. Brofaromine was discontinued quite late in development. Moclobemide is a potent but selective and reversible inhibitor of MAO-A. It has no other significant biochemical effects. It increases brain amines but in a short-lasting way. At therapeutic dose levels (300–600 mg/day), moclobemide potentiates oral tyramine four to seven fold, which is too low to be of any clinical significance as it would be difficult to eat sufficient cheese, say, for a pressor effect. Unlike other MAOIs, moclobemide has little effect on sleep patterns.

Moclobemide is rapidly and completely absorbed after oral administration and is extensively distributed into the tissues. It is metabolised by the liver and neither age nor kidney disease affect this.

Moclobemide is superior to placebo in the treatment of patients with major depression and has proved equally effective across various subtypes of depressives. It seems of similar efficacy to standard TCAs but is often more activating. Comparisons with SSRIs are too few to draw conclusions from.

The drug is well-tolerated (Table 9.1), nausea and insomnia being the only side-effects recorded more frequently than with placebo. It has no consistent effect on blood pressure nor does oedema seem to be a problem. The elderly tolerate the drug well. It has few if any anticholinergic effects, unlike the TCAs and the earlier MAOIs. Nor does it cause restlessness. It is considerably less toxic in overdose than its predecessors. Dietary precautions have been judged not to be necessary but it is recommended that the drug be taken after meals to minimise any possible tyramine interaction.

Moclobemide is an interesting introduction with a much improved risk/benefit ratio to the old MAOIs. It might even be acceptable in depressed schizophrenic patients who were actually made worse by the older drugs. Its progress in the crowded antidepressant market will be watched with great interest. In particular, predictors of response should be sought in large-scale post-marketing studies.

PSYCHOLOGICAL EFFECTS OF ANTIDEPRESSANTS

Depression itself may have profound effects on psychological functioning and therefore performance and cognition. Tiredness, lassitude, poor concentration and lack of interest or motivation are common features of the disorder. At its most severe, sufferers may be either so retarded or so anguished that they are able to accomplish nothing. The effects of drugs are therefore related to the condition.

Effects of Tricyclic Antidepressants in Healthy Volunteers

The effects of antidepressants have been much less systematically investigated than those of benzodiazepines. However, since the advent of newer compounds and an increase in the prescription rate, interest has grown in the comparative effects. In general, small doses of sedative compounds, like amitriptyline, exert a calming effect but as the dose is increased, there may be marked sedation associated with widespread performance decrement in healthy volunteers. This is true of both older and newer compounds (trazodone) and has been found after both acute and repeated doses. Amitriptyline has been the most studied especially in comparison with newer antidepressants because of its sedative action. In comparison to several other TCAs, amitriptyline has been shown to consistently impair both psychomotor and attentional tasks. Other sedative compounds like trazodone and mianserin have been shown to impair performance but the decrement is less. Amitriptyline has also been found to have effects on cognitive functioning. While the psychomotor effects seem to be largely accounted for by sedation, the effects on memory have been attributed to its anticholinergic action. Imipramine has been shown to produce some measurable cognitive impairment but other TCAs with less anticholinergic action (clomipramine, desipramine) have not.

Effects of TCAs in Depressed Patients

The psychological effects of TCAs in depressed patients are much less clear but the weight of evidence suggests a beneficial rather than a detrimental effect. Although some studies have shown cognitive impairment after a single dose, this seems to remit rapidly. Most studies have used higher doses and longer time intervals (two to eight weeks) than those in healthy volunteers. Thus tolerance to the drug may be compounded by improvement in clinical state. There is in fact some evidence that depressed patients show improvement in memory tasks after repeated doses of imipramine despite no noticeable improvement in mood. It may be therefore that cognition sequentially improves after sleep and appetite along with concentration and attention and before the lifting of depressed mood.

It therefore seems unlikely that TCAs lead to any relevant impairment of memory functions in depressed patients, especially when they are used within an individual therapeutic programme of gradually increased doses. However, those with anticholinergic effects, like amitriptyline, should be avoided in the elderly as there is some evidence that the effects on secondary memory increase with age.

Effects of SSRIs

In general, SSRIs exert minimal effects on measures of performance and cognition despite some subjective sedation. Only supratherapeutic doses have been shown to have any detrimental effect in healthy volunteers. Repeated dose studies in depressed patients have also failed to show any deficits and improvement in cognitive functioning has been related to a lessening of depressed mood.

Effects of RIMAs

The advent of the reversible, predominately MAO-A inhibitors, has led to studies of their effects on performance and cognition compared to other antidepressants. Studies of single doses of moclobemide in healthy volunteers have failed to reveal any significant impairment on either subjective ratings or memory functions. In one study, moclobemide was shown to restore mental efficiency which had been impaired by the administration of a challenge dose of scopolamine. Other studies have revealed no effect on higher cognitive functions and only minimal effects on RT or vigilance tasks. Repeated dose studies in both healthy volunteers and depressed patients confirm these promising results and indicate that this group of drugs may have some cognitive enhancing properties in both elderly subjects and young depressed patients. However more studies in depressed patients are required.

OTHER DRUGS USED AS ANTIDEPRESSANTS

Several reports, including controlled studies, have attested to the useful antidepressant properties of *antipsychotic drugs* in low dosage. These claims have involved flupenthixol and sulpiride in particular. The mode of action is postulated to involve presynaptic blockade of noradrenaline and dopamine receptors resulting in increased synthesis and release. At higher, antipsychotic doses, postsynaptic blockade occurs and attenuates the antidepressant response. Clinically, flupenthixol and sulpiride can be useful in treating otherwise refractory patients, although some observers have noted that the response may wane over the ensuing six months.

Benzodiazepines have been used to treat depression, and one, alprazolam, underwent trials for this indication. Although some symptomatic relief of anxiety and agitation may be helpful to some patients, in general effects on depression are usually minimal. Indeed, by lessening the anxiety and thereby uncovering the depression, benzodiazepines may appear to make some patients worse.

Amine precursors have long been suggested as antidepressants either alone or as adjuncts to other treatment. *L-tryptophan* administration increases brain serotonin in animals and has useful antidepressant actions in man. The clearest evidence suggests that it potentiates other antidepressants, especially those acting on serotonin mechanisms such as clomipramine. L-tryptophan was available to treat depression but had to be withdrawn from the market when a curious untoward effect was noted. This comprised a change in the blood cells (eosinophilia) and muscle pain (myalgia). It was traced to a contaminant which was eliminated, and the drug has been made available again.

TREATMENT ISSUES

Maintenance and Prophylaxis

Relapse can be defined as a return of symptoms satisfying the criteria for a depressive disorder which occurs within six months of apparent recovery from a depressive episode. Surveys have suggested that the total duration of a depressive episode averages 6–9 months in out-patients and 9–12 months in those who require admission to hospital at some time. As recovery takes up to three and six months respectively, this leaves about six months 'at risk' of relapse.

Recently, there has been increasing awareness that as depressive episodes last up to a year, treatment must also be directed towards maintenance and not just short-term efficacy. It is now clear from a series of trials that anti-depressants given for only six to eight weeks are an inadequate treatment. If they are discontinued prematurely, about half of patients will relapse in the ensuing six months. If they are continued, less than a quarter of patients will relapse back into depression. This has led to the generally-accepted recommendation that antidepressants should be continued for at least four to six months after apparent recovery. Added to the initial course of treatment, this means that the total exposure to an antidepressant should routinely exceed six months. In the licensing of new drugs, longer-term studies are becoming increasingly important both to estimate effectiveness in preventing relapse and in minimising the risk of possible long-term toxicity.

Recurrence is the onset of symptoms meeting depressive disorder criteria which occur after six months of apparent recovery from a depressive disorder. This may be 9–12 months after the onset of the previous episode but usually the inter-episode interval is longer, averaging three years.

The use of antidepressants to prevent further episodes of illness has become increasingly common. With bipolar illnesses, lithium is usually the drug of choice (see Chapter 10). However, many psychiatrists prefer antidepressant therapy for unipolar depressives. Because of the timescale of the appropriate studies, few drugs have been evaluated in this way. The evidence is strongest for imipramine which reduces recurrences, as compared with placebo, to half or even a third. Other TCAs and newer drugs have also been subject to some studies. Thus, the usefulness of fluoxetine, paroxetine, sertraline, and citalopram has been shown. The good tolerability of the SSRIs makes them attractive for long-term use apart from their expense.

Use in Primary Care

Depression is a common condition, most patients presenting first in primary care settings. As well as major depressive disorder, the syndromes commonly seen include minor depressive episodes and lifelong fluctuating mild depression. Brief recurrent depression is also a mode of presentation. Most depressives present for help in general practice but there is concern that in up to half of such patients the diagnosis is missed, at least at the initial consultation.

The management of depression combines psychosocial management with drug therapy as appropriate. Antidepressants are effective in patients whose illnesses satisfy the criteria for major depressive disorder but most need full doses (equivalent to at least 125 mg/day imipramine) for adequate response. At the mild end of the clinical range antidepressant therapy is not effective. A patient may have moderate depression but the condition seems reactive to life-circumstances: antidepressants are still indicated.

GPs have their own predilections concerning the choice of antidepressant but often use a sedative drug such as dothiepin. It is often given at night to act as an hypnotic as well. GPs often terminate treatment rather too early, particularly when the patient complains of persistent side-effects.

The Treatment of Refractory Depression

This is very much the province of the psychiatrist who sees depressed patients who have failed to respond to one or more of the standard therapies as prescribed by the GP. Sometimes the dosage is insufficient but many patients respond inadequately if at all to what should have been an effective drug regimen. Consequently, the psychiatrist encounters a biased sample of patients.

One cause of apparent non-response is poor compliance. This important factor is discussed in Chapter 3. The delay to onset of improvement, the burden of side-effects, particularly in the elderly, and the despair, despondency, and lack of motivation which permeate the depressed person all militate against adherence to the prescribed drug dosage and frequency. Gaining the confidence of the patient is important and education can be crucial in modifying the patient's attitudes towards accepting medication.

Organic factors can render a depressive patient refractory to treatment. Hepatitis, viral pneumonia, infective mononucleosis (glandular fever) and brucellosis (undulant fever) are infections which can be associated with persistent depression. Cancer of the pancreas, and endocrine disturbances are other causes. In the elderly, early dementia may be difficult to differentiate from depression: indeed, the two may co-exist. Lesions in the brain such as epileptic foci, tumours and infarcts from strokes are other possible causes. Parkinsonism and multiple sclerosis are neurological conditions particularly liable to induce resistant depression. A variety of drugs can be implicated: antihypertensive drugs, corticosteroids and perhaps oral contraceptives. Abuse of alcohol and other substances is a common complicating factor.

The management of resistant depression occupies much of the typical specialist psychiatrist's time. Generally speaking a series of antidepressants is used, each with the dosage pushed as high as tolerated or practical. Lithium may be added to boost the response or L-tryptophan or buspirone used as an adjunct. It may help to monitor plasma drug concentrations, at least to check compliance. The use of MAOIs will probably increase with the introduction of moclobemide. Unfortunately, no guarantee of success can be made to any patient so it is vitally important to retain his/her confidence in the prescriber.

PSYCHOLOGICAL THERAPY OF DEPRESSION

In mild depressive disorder, drug treatment has less to offer and psychosocial factors assume greater importance. Often simple supportive therapy or brief interventions targeted at modifying these factors (Table 9.2) and administered by a GP or practice counsellor may suffice. Marital therapy or brief focal therapy based on a psychodynamic model may also be helpful in mild depression but moderate depression requires therapy using a more structured approach administered by a trained practitioner. The two most established psychological therapies for depression are cognitive therapy and inter-personal therapy.

Table 9.2 Treatment of mild depression

---

1. Support
2. Life-style advice
3. Empathic listening
4. Increase of activities
5. Problem solving

Cognitive Therapy

Cognitive therapy (CT) is based on the cognitive model (Chapter 2) which suggests that experience leads to people to form beliefs about themselves, the world and the future (cognitive triad). In depression dysfunctional beliefs may be activated by a critical incident leading to negative thoughts. The aim of therapy is to enable patients to question their own negative automatic thoughts and then challenge and correct the faulty beliefs underlying them. As various behavioural techniques may be used to test beliefs, CT is often referred to as cognitive behaviour therapy (CBT). Many studies have established the efficacy of CT or CBT compared to no treatment and some have shown it to be superior to less structured treatments such as client-centred or psychodynamic therapies. Some studies have attempted to evaluate the effectiveness of cognitive therapy compared to treatment with tricyclics. These studies often suffer from methodological weaknesses such as inadequate dose levels, a lack of placebo control or inappropriate selection of patient groups for drug treatment, which may bias the results towards a favourable outcome for cognitive therapy. Nevertheless, the general conclusion can be drawn that cognitive therapy is roughly comparable to TCAs in the acute treatment of moderate depression. The data on long-term outcome are less clear. When an acute period of treatment with TCAs or CT is terminated and patients are followed up for one to two years post treatment, patients who have been treated with CT show a significantly better outcome and a lower rate of attrition. However, the claim that CT always leads to a more favourable outcome than TCA treatment must be tempered by the contention that an inadequate period of drug treatment has been administered. CT certainly seems to be as effective as maintenance or continuation treatment with TCAs and it seems to be the only current treatment which may provide continued benefit after termination of therapy. Relapse rates of patients with recurrent depression are high and so any treatment indicating continued improvement must be a preferred option. However, the number of trained practitioners is still limited and CT requires not only good rapport but the active collaboration of the patient. There is insufficient evidence to recommend its sole use in severe depression although the combined use of drug and psychological treatment is advocated for severe, complex or non-responsive cases. In more severe depression, patients receiving cognitive therapy are at more risk of relapse and may need longer courses of treatment.

Interpersonal Therapy

Interpersonal therapy is based on the assumption that the precipitating cause of depression usually occurs in an interpersonal context. Treatment focuses on improving the quality of the current interpersonal functioning of the patient so that they can recognise problems. Interpersonal therapy has been shown to be roughly comparable to TCAs in the acute treatment of moderate depression and to help to prolong remission when administered as maintenance therapy.

Combined Treatment of Depression

Several studies have purported to examine the combination of TCA and cognitive therapies in the treatment of depression but again methodological weaknesses abound, reducing the number of studies from which a conclusion can be drawn. Although it cannot be said that the combination of TCAs and CT is clearly superior with regard to acute response to either treatment administered alone, most of the studies do report positive results and non-significant trends favour the combined treatments on nearly every relevant measure. Additional studies with larger sample sizes could give definitive answers. When long-term outcome is evaluated, the evidence indicates that cognitive and interpersonal therapy, either following or in combination with TCA treatment, both lower relapse rate. Unfortunately, because of drop-outs due to attrition and additional treatment, follow-up studies involve only small numbers of patients who have both completed and responded to the study treatment and so such results cannot be generalised to the bulk of patients entering therapy. Follow-up times are generally not long enough to determine if this apparent preventative capacity has any prophylactic effect against new episodes.

Predictors of Treatment Response

Very few studies have attempted to predict which patients will respond to which treatment. One large collaborative study (NIMH) indicated that drug treatment was superior to cognitive therapy in severe depression involving impairment of functioning, but a further breakdown of the results showed this to be true for only one of the three sites and the execution of the cognitive therapy at this site has therefore been questioned. Another study looked at significant life stressors but found that pre-treatment psychosocial stress scores did not predict response to cognitive therapy as opposed to imipramine. In the same way, biological markers do not seem to predict response to treatment with antidepressant drugs. Recent studies have focused on personality traits and the possibility that these variables might predict treatment response or selection. Beck (1976) described two personality traits important in depression: sociotropy (a concern with rejection by others) and autonomy (a concern with personal failure). There is some preliminary evidence that patients high on autonomy and low on sociotropy show more response to antidepressant drug treatment. Other studies have tried to link Cloninger's temperament variables (novelty seeking, harm avoidance and reward dependence) to response to antidepressant drug treatment (Cloninger, 1987). Although the relationships between traits was too complex to be discussed here, temperament did have more predictive value than any of the clinical variables measured. This area is likely to expand as both cognitive interventions and SSRIs make inroads in the treatment of personality disorder. It should be noted here that no comparisons have yet been published of SSRIs or RIMAs compared to or combined with cognitive therapy in the treatment of depression.

SUMMARY

Depression is a common condition which is often overlooked but which may cause impaired work and social functioning. There is evidence that mono-amine neurotransmitters, in particular serotonin, are deficient in people with depression. The tricyclic antidepressants were the first effective drugs to be used in the treatment of depression. There is no evidence that newer antidepressants such as selective serotonin re-uptake inhibitors are more effective but they have a different profile of unwanted effects which may make them better tolerated, thus improving compliance. Monoamine oxidase inhibitors are much less used because of their potential toxicity but the recent introduction of a safe, reversible inhibitor of monoamine oxidase may prove to be a popular addition. The therapeutic response to all antidepressants is delayed for two to three weeks and depressive mood is often one of the last elements of the disorder to respond to treatment. The two established psychological therapies for depression are cognitive therapy and inter-personal therapy. Cognitive therapy seems to be as effective as maintenance treatment with TCAs and it is the only current treatment which may provide continued benefit after termination of therapy. The combination of psychological and drug therapy seems to lower relapse rate.

FURTHER READING

Allain, H., Lieury, A., Brunet-Bourgin, F. et al. (1992) Antidepressants and cognition: comparative effects of moclobemide, viloxazine and maprotiline. *Psychopharmacology* **106**, S56–S61.
Beck, A.T. (1976) *Cognitive Therapy and the Emotional Disorders*. International Universities Press, New York.
Beck, A.T., Rush, A.J., Shaw, B.F. and Emery, G. (1979) *Cognitive Therapy of Depression: A Treatment Manual*. Guilford Press, New York.

Brown, W.A. and Khan, A. (1994) Which depressed patients should receive antidepressants? *CNS Drugs* **1**, 341–347.

Cloninger, C.R. (1987) A systematic method of clinical description and classification of personality variants. *Archives of General Psychiatry* **44**, 573–588.

Davidson, J., Zung, W.W.K. and Walker, J.I. (1984) Practical aspects of MAO inhibitor therapy. *Journal of Clinical Psychiatry* **45 (Sec.2)**, 81–84.

Elkin, I., Shea, T., Watkins, J.T. et al. (1989) National Institute of Mental Health Treatment of Depression Collaborative Research Program. *Archives of General Psychiatry* **46**, 971–982.

Fitton, A., Faulds, D. and Goa, K.L. (1992) Moclobemide. A review of its pharmacological properties and therapeutic use in depressive illness. *Drugs* **43**, 561–596.

Freemantle, N., House, A., Song, F., Mason, J.M. and Sheldon, T.A. (1994) Prescribing selective serotonin reuptake inhibitors as strategy for prevention of suicide. *British Medical Journal* **309**, 249–253.

Greden, J.F. (1993) Antidepressant maintenance medications: when to discontinue and how to stop. *Journal of Clinical Psychiatry* **54 (suppl. 8)**, 39–45.

Guscott, R. and Grof, P. (1991) The clinical meaning of refractory depression: a review for the clinician. *American Journal of Psychiatry* **148**, 695–704.

Hobi, V., Gastpar, M., Gastpar, G., Gilsdorf, U., Kielholz, P. and Schwarz, E. (1982) Driving ability of depressive patients under antidepressants. *Journal of International Medical Research* **10**, 65–81.

Hollon, S.D., Shelton, R.C. and Davis, D.D. (1993) Cognitive therapy for depression: conceptual issues and clinical efficacy. *Journal of Consulting and Clinical Psychology* **61**, 270–275.

Judd, L.L., Squire, L.R., Butters, N., Salmon, D.P. and Paller, K.A. (1987) Effects of psychotropic drugs on cognition and memory in normal humans and animals. In *Psychopharmacology: The Third Generation of Progress* (Meltzer, H.Y., ed.). Raven Press, New York, pp. 1467–1475.

Klerman, G.L., Weissman, M.M., Rounsaville, B.J. et al. (1984) *Interpersonal Psychotherapy of Depression*. Basic Books, New York.

Kuhn, R. (1958) The treatment of depressive states with G22355 (imipramine hydrochloride). *American Journal of Psychiatry* **115**, 459–463.

Kupfer, D.J. (1991) Long-term treatment of depression. *Journal of Clinical Psychiatry* **52**:5 (suppl.), 28–34.

Meterissian, G.B. and Bradwejn, J. (1989) Comparative studies on the efficacy of psychotherapy, pharmacotherapy, and their combination in depression: was adequate pharmacotherapy provided? *Journal of Clinical Psychopharmacology* **9**, 334–339.

Montgomery, S.A., Henry, J., McDonald, G. et al. (1994) Selective serotonin re-uptake inhibitors: meta-analysis of discontinuation rates. *International Clinical Psychopharmacology* **9**, 47–53.

Pancheri, P., Delle Chiaie, R., Donnini, M. et al. (1994) Effects of moclobemide on depressive symptoms and cognitive performance in a geriatric population: a controlled comparative study versus imipramine. *Clinical Neuropharmacology* **17: 1** (suppl.), S58–S73.

Paykel, E.S. and Priest, R.G. (1992) Recognition and management of depression in general practice: consensus statement. *British Medical Journal* **305**, 1198–1202.

Rudorfer, M.V. and Potter, W.Z. (1989) Antidepressants. A comparative review of the clinical pharmacology and therapeutic use of the 'newer' versus the 'older' drugs. *Drugs* **37**, 713–738.

Sotsky, S.M., Glass, D.R., Shea, M.T. (1991) Patient predictors of response to psychotherapy and pharmacotherapy: findings in the NIMH Treatment of Depression Collaborative Research Program. *American Journal of Psychiatry* **148**, 997–1008.

Thompson, P.J. (1991) Antidepressants and memory: a review. *Human Psychopharmacology* **6**, 79–90.

Thompson, P.J. and Trimble, M.R. (1982) Non-MAOI antidepressant drugs and cognitive functions: a review. *Psychological Medicine* **12**, 539–548.

Wells, K.B., Burnam, A, Rogers, W., Hays, R. and Camp, P. (1992) The course of depression in adult outpatients. Results from the Medical Outcomes Study. *Archives of General Psychiatry* **49**, 788–794.

Chapter 10

TREATMENT OF MANIA AND BIPOLAR DISORDER

In this chapter, the treatment of mania and bipolar disorder is outlined. The use of lithium therapy is described in detail and both the therapeutic and unwanted effects are delineated. Alternatives to lithium are discussed as well as the uses of lithium in other disorders.

Mania indicates a disturbance in mood which is opposite to that of depression. Mood is persistently elevated and energy and activity levels are increased over a period of time, without relationship to events. The symptoms tend to be opposite to those of depression (Figure 10.1), thus self-esteem is inflated and there is an increase in energy, reducing the need for sleep. Agitation and poor concentration may be a feature of both conditions, but in mania they are accompanied by overactivity and marked distractibility. Behavioural changes are marked and may cause distress to relatives and danger to the patient. Severe mania causes marked impairment in occupational and social functioning. Grandiose ideas may develop into delusions and irritability and suspiciousness into delusions of persecution and episodes of aggression or violence. A less severe form of mania which does not cause the same degree of occupational or social impairment is known as hypomania. This is often seen as patients either develop or recover from mania.

Bipolar disorder is characterised by repeated episodes of mood disturbance where this disturbance may sometimes be elevated mood and increased activity levels (mania) and at other times lowered mood and decreased activity levels (depression). The depressive episodes are generally indistinguishable from episodes of unipolar depression. There is recovery between episodes.

LITHIUM

Lithium is a simple metallic cation, number three in the Periodic Table, after hydrogen and helium. It is widely found in nature and forms complex mineral salts. Lithium salts, themselves, were used in the 19th century in the treatment

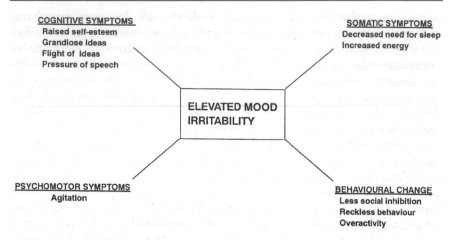

Figure 10.1   Features of mania

of gout, some forms of mental disorder, and other maladies. These 'Lithia' tablets were soon found to have toxic effects on the heart, and fell into disuse. Lithium salts were reintroduced in the 1940s as a taste substitute in salt-free (low sodium chloride) diets but were again discarded because of cardiotoxicity. Eventually lithium was found to be a useful therapeutic and preventative agent, with acceptable risks if properly administered and monitored. As with any effective psychotropic compound, lithium has been tried in a wide range of psychiatric conditions with varying degrees of success.

Pharmacokinetics

Lithium is one of the few psychotropic drugs whose blood level is monitored routinely. This is because the so-called 'therapeutic index' is low, i.e. the toxic level is uncomfortably close to the therapeutic.

Lithium is well-absorbed and sustained release preparations which smooth out the peaks of absorption have become standard. Lithium takes some time to distribute uniformly in the body and the brain. Lithium cannot be metabolised but it is excreted through the kidney into the urine. Here it reaches local concentrations much higher than in the rest of the body. Excretion of lithium is closely dependent on that of sodium: if sodium intake is restricted, e.g. a faddy diet, or sodium excretion increased, e.g. with a diuretic drug, lithium excretion is reduced and it may accumulate in the body reaching toxic levels.

It is essential to monitor serum lithium concentrations regularly. On initiation of therapy, estimations are usually taken weekly for the first four to six weeks and then every three to six weeks thereafter, or less frequently in trustworthy, well-stabilised patients. Any change in dose, especially an increase, must also be carefully monitored. The usual range aimed at for prevention of affective episodes is about 0.6–1.2 millimoles per litre but higher levels may be needed to treat acute hypomanic relapses. Toxicity generally occurs above 2 mmol/l. The estimations are a complement to clinical observation and not a substitute. The tendency over the years has been to edge the usual dosage range downwards. The blood sample is taken at a standardised time, just before the dose after the longest inter-dose interval during the 24 hours.

Pharmacology

Lithium, despite being chemically simple, has a complex and only partially understood pharmacology. It competes with other cations but also has actions in its own right. One important action is on the second messenger system, phosphoinositol. Evidence has accrued over the years linking some at least of the therapeutic effects of lithium to an effect on serotonin systems, sensitising them.

Therapeutic Effects

Lithium is used primarily to treat manic and hypomanic patients and to prevent attacks of mania and depression in patients with recurrent affective disorders. Its efficacy in schizo-affective disorder is less well-established. A wide range of other conditions in which lithium has been tried with varying success include the acute treatment of depressive illness, epilepsy, various forms of aggression, alcoholism, schizophrenia, and movement disorders.

Treatment of Mania and Hypomania

Antipsychotic medication is the other type of treatment widely used in this indication and it is often combined with lithium. Uncontrolled trials suggested that about 80% of manic patients settle down on lithium. Controlled trials confirmed this efficacy, usually with comparisons to an active treatment such as chlorpromazine or haloperidol. However, the number of placebo-controlled trials is quite low. Lithium takes up to a week for its efficacy to become established and this is too long to wait in the more severely ill patients. In the more mildly affected patients, symptom control is adequate quite early on and the patients often prefer lithium's effects to the over-sedation induced by antipsychotic medication.

The combination of haloperidol and lithium is commonly used despite some reports of enhanced toxicity. Concern over these reports appears to have subsided although careful monitoring remains essential and dosage should be conservative.

Treatment of Depression

The earliest reports suggested that lithium was ineffective in treating acutely depressed patients. Later reports began to question this negative finding and, more recently, it has become apparent that bipolar manic-depressive patients in a depressive phase may often respond quite well to the administration of lithium alone. A further series of studies has suggested that lithium is useful in the treatment of refractory depressives, usually added as an adjunct to a standard antidepressant, a TCA or an SSRI. Response is usually seen within a few days.

Prevention of Affective Disorders

This use of lithium was originally a matter of great controversy, mainly because of the inadequate design of some of the earlier studies. Establishing efficacy in a long-term indication is difficult and arduous, but essential because the drug will be taken by patients for a long time with the risk of chronic toxicity.

The situation was eventually resolved by the completion of several studies in which patients meeting criteria for recurrent affective disorder, unipolar and/ or bipolar, were allocated randomly and prospectively to several years of treatment with lithium or placebo (or in some trials, a TCA). The relapse rate, often defined operationally as hospital admission, was used as the main outcome variable. By and large, lithium significantly decreases the number of hypomanic relapses, and in some patients the effect is dramatic, transforming the patient's life from a series of disruptive and embarrassing manic excursions to an even tenor of existence. The effect on depressive episodes is less dramatic and in unipolar patients at least no better than that of long-term antidepressant maintenance. Not only are the number of affective episodes lessened by lithium but the severity of those that do occur is greatly attenuated. This has given rise to the suggestion that lithium may not actually *prevent* episodes but by treating them as they ensue it *reduces* their severity to mild degrees or to a subclinical level.

Bipolar patients with rapidly alternating cycles, weeks rather than months or years, often do poorly on lithium and other medications such as carbamazepine are often preferred. However, these patients are often notoriously difficult to treat and lithium is still worth trying. Mania of late age of onset also responds poorly.

Prediction of Response

Several trials have attempted to distinguish predictors of good response to lithium in the prophylaxis of manic-depressive illness. Early failure to respond adequately, e.g. in the first year of lithium treatment, predicts that later response will also be poor. A wide range of other factors such as age, age of onset, retardation, family history of bipolar illness, suicidal intent, and neuroticism, have all been studied but with no conclusive results. Psychological factors such as MMPI profile, Eysenck Personality Questionnaire scores, obsessionality and pre-morbid lability have also failed to provide clear prognostic indicators. Nor have biological predictors such as thyroid function, serotonin transport into the blood platelet or platelet monoamine oxidase levels proved helpful. Therefore, the only way of predicting response is a trial of lithium therapy; those who do well will continue to do well.

Indications for Prophylactic Treatment

It is appropriate to start prophylaxis if a patient is expected to suffer two further episodes in the subsequent five years. In retrospective terms, the criteria translate into the presence of one episode in the previous five years in unipolar depressives, in the previous four years in bipolars, and in the previous three years in schizo-affective disorder. The general guidelines are that prophylactic treatment should be started in unipolar depression after three episodes, one being in the past five years, in addition to the current one; in bipolar illness, lithium should be started after the second episode.

The possible effects of lithium maintenance on the high mortality associated with affective disorder, mainly from suicide, have been evaluated. Essentially, the data indicate that in patients stabilised on lithium, mortality, as one indicator of morbidity, is reduced. This effect cannot be seen in cohorts evaluated prospectively on an intent-to-treat basis because of the early drop-out of many patients at particularly high risk because of the refractory nature of their illness.

Other Indications

Schizo-affective disorders combine some of the features of schizophrenia and some of those of affective disorders. Both 'schizomanic' and 'schizodepressive' episodes can occur. The latter are hard to distinguish from depressive episodes occurring in schizophrenic patients. Furthermore, schizo-affective symptoms often become more clearly schizophrenic in type as episodes recur. In general, however, the prognosis is better than in schizophrenia. Lithium has been shown to be useful as prophylaxis in schizo-affective patients, but the manic episodes are usually better controlled than the depressive.

Lithium therapy has been tried in patients with alcohol problems. As alcoholism may be secondary to affective changes, lithium may be helpful in carefully selected patients. The therapeutic effect is mainly secondary to a stabilisation of mood, but a primary effect on the urge to drink may also operate.

Another indication, a rather ill-defined one, for which lithium has been advocated is in the management of hostile and violent patients. Controlled studies have suggested some lessening of aggression in antisocial (sociopathic) prisoners and also in patients with learning difficulties prone to unprovoked aggression and temper tantrums.

Unwanted Effects

Acute Effects

Nausea is a common side-effect and it is frequently accompanied by loose bowel movements (Table 10.1). Although these effects are a nuisance, they tend to wane over a few weeks and do not usually result in discontinuation of the medication. Another common side-effect is a fine tremor of the fingers which can be obtrusive in patients whose work entails precise movements. This symptom tends to persist. Increased production of urine (polyuria) is dose-dependent and results from lithium's blockade of the regulatory antidiuretic hormone in the kidney. It can occur at night and actually disturbs sleep because of repeated trips to void urine. If calorie-rich drinks are used to slake thirst, weight increase can be even greater than it usually is on lithium.

Chronic Effects

Tremor, polyuria and weight gain often persist into the long-term. Benign swelling of the thyroid gland (goitre) may occur, usually with depression of

Table 10.1   Side-effects of lithium

Neurological	Tremor
Gastrointestinal	Nausea
	Diarrhoea
Renal	Polyuria → Polydipsia
Thyroid function	Goitre
	Hypothyroidism
Weight gain	

thyroid function (hypothyroidism). It is not common but should be borne in mind especially if some apparent retardation ensues in the patient. Patients with low or borderline thyroid function before instituting lithium are at particular risk so it is customary to assess thyroid function beforehand. If hypothyroidism does supervene it can be treated simply with thyroid hormone supplements.

Long-term effects on the kidney were described 10–15 years ago and caused some alarm. However, careful evaluation of thousands of patients has failed to confirm any link between lithium treatment and kidney damage. Nevertheless, unnecessarily high lithium concentrations in the body, and hence the kidney, are best avoided. Patients should be screened for adequate kidney function before starting lithium.

Other long-term symptoms include poor memory, indigestion, aches and pains, slurred speech and rashes including the worsening or precipitation of psoriasis and acne. Lithium should be avoided during pregnancy as there is clear evidence of heart malformations in a significant proportion of the babies. Lactating mothers should stop breast-feeding their babies if lithium is indicated after childbirth.

Toxic Effects

Vomiting and diarrhoea, increased tremor, muscular weakness, drowsiness, unsteadiness and slurred speech are all signs that the safe dosage has been exceeded. More serious effects include twitching, disorientation, restlessness, confusion, fits and eventually coma and death. The kidneys may cease functioning so that dialysis is needed. Even with recovery from severe toxicity, brain damage may be permanent with particular effects on the cerebellum resulting in movement disorders.

Psychological Effects

The practice of prescribing lithium has changed in recent years. It has been recognised that lower doses are equally effective and a reduction in dose has resulted in a reduced frequency and intensity of side-effects which has been reflected in effects on psychological performance. The introduction of newer slow release formulations has also added to this improved side-effect profile.

Effects in Healthy Volunteers

Several studies have looked at the effects of lithium on normal, non-pathological mood. Older studies reported increased feelings of tiredness and malaise but more recent studies have shown no effect on mood and no increased reporting of physical complaints after an acute dose. Subjects were generally unable to discriminate between lithium and placebo. Other studies have examined the effects of repeated doses. These studies have used doses at the lower end of the therapeutic range in order to minimise side-effects while looking for a mood stabilisation effect of lithium over a period of several weeks. Lithium was found to be well tolerated with no overall effects on mood. Mood variability tended to decrease as a function of time in study rather than treatment status. However there were large interindividual differences and there was evidence of both dysphoria and mood stabilisation in some subjects. It is likely that initial status is a very important factor.

Older studies reported that lithium produced both psychomotor and cognitive impairment. Such effects were small and were attributed to a slowing in the rate of central information processing as accuracy was not affected. It has also been suggested that the motor side-effects of lithium (tremor, ataxia) may have contributed to these deficits. Effects on various performance tasks including vigilance and tracking have not been replicated in recent studies and no evidence has been found of smooth pursuit eye movement dysfunction after two weeks of treatment. Neither has performance on cognitive tasks such as syntactic reasoning, free recall or recognition memory shown any impairment after acute or repeated doses in recent studies. However some more subtle effects have been shown to emerge after repeated doses. Subjects are more likely to make errors of commission or intrusion on recall tasks after one week's treatment. The additional words produced are appropriate to the task stimuli but consist of material which has not been presented during the test session and so this has been described as a 'cognitive blurring'. This lack of clarity of what is remembered may be reflected in subjective memory complaints.

Effects in Patients

Studies which have compared mood states and day-to-day variability of mood between euthymic bipolar patients treated with lithium and control subjects have generally found variability to be lower among the treated patients. This result may be due to bipolar patients' experience of much more extreme moods leading to a narrowing of what they perceive as normal or euthymic. A similar problem attends subjective complaints of being slowed down, less attentive and more forgetful which have been noted after lithium treatment. Such complaints are difficult to interpret if the subjective comparison is with a manic state. Subjective memory complaints of patients maintained on lithium do not differ from those of patients on antidepressant medication and it has been suggested that they are linked to underlying psychopathology such as depression. This is lent some support by correlations which have been found between subjective memory complaints and scores on depression scales. However, such beliefs should be addressed as they may be rooted in subtle memory changes and may affect compliance. One study has attempted systematically to answer the subjective complaint of reduced creativity. Of 24 artists with bipolar disorder currently being treated with lithium, six reported lower creativity, another six no change and 12 that they created more and in some cases better during treatment. There are then large individual differences in subjective effects.

There are few controlled studies of the effects of lithium on performance of patients and contradictory conclusions abound. Although there is some evidence that reaction time and other driving skills may be slowed, these changes are usually very small after long-term treatment and accuracy does not seem to be affected. Patients should be cautioned as when taking numerous other drugs. It has been claimed that lithium affects smooth pursuit eye movements but a study among patients with their first episode of bipolar disorder found no difference between those taking and not taking lithium. There was no further change after 10 months treatment. It is concluded that any such effect could be due to a chronic illness or to prior medication and is not a direct effect of lithium treatment. Studies of cognitive function have shown no effects on immediate or short-term retrieval and no evidence of cognitive impairment in cross-sectional studies comparing patients with bipolar illness treated with lithium (for over two years) with those untreated or on a tricyclic antidepressant. Nor was there any difference between patients receiving short-term or long-term lithium treatment. A longitudinal study has found memory test scores for both verbal and visual material to remain remarkably stable over six years. Evidence for lithium producing some memory impairment in patients comes from studies which have manipulated lithium status in the same patients. Discontinuation of chronic lithium (average treatment period of nine years) generally resulted in improved performance and reinstatement led to a subsequent decline on measures of long-term storage and retrieval. Unfortunately no pre-lithium assessments were carried out.

In conclusion, the newer formulations and lower doses of lithium which are used currently produce much less impairment than previous regimens. There is no evidence of widespread cognitive impairment and, although some slowing and subtle memory changes may be produced, these seem to be readily reversible on termination of treatment.

Use of Lithium

The prescription of lithium requires expertise and experience. For this reason some mental health services have set up special lithium clinics where patients can be treated by specialists. Regular monitoring of serum lithium levels is available and thyroid function can be tested regularly. Experience is built up on when to recommend lithium, how to administer it and how long to continue. Counselling can be given to the patient, to help convince of the need for, and the value of prophylactic long-term lithium therapy. Sometimes the patient regrets losing his/her hypomanic episodes which are the times when he/she feels best. Attending a clinic with other patients encourages compliance and lifts morale. It can even provide an informal sort of psychotherapy. Standardised records are often kept so that the patient's progress, or lack of response, can be followed in a more graphic way than the usual hospital records. Monitoring serum levels emphasises to the patient the need for careful compliance. Finally, the decision about whether and when to try to stop therapy can be made on the basis of a full knowledge of the patient's previous history.

CARBAMAZEPINE

This drug is an example of a mood-stabilising treatment which has been developed by research clinicians, and which is now quite widely used as a mood regulator, but for which insufficient systematic data are available for formal licensing for this indication. Carbamazepine has been used for many years in the treatment of some forms of epilepsy (see p. 217) and of trigeminal neuralgia, a spasmodic painful affliction of the face. It is chemically related to imipramine.

Both uncontrolled and controlled studies suggest useful efficacy in the treatment of manic and hypomanic episodes. Its efficacy has also been assessed in the prophylaxis of affective disorders. In general, it is less effective than lithium but may be worth trying especially in rapid cyclers. Other conditions in which some efficacy of carbamazepine has been claimed include schizo-affective disorder and aggressive episodes in schizophrenic patients.

Carbamazepine has a range of unwanted effects including drowsiness, dizziness, nausea and double-vision. Drug interactions are common. Carbamazepine's level in the blood can be monitored to maintain the patient's dosage such that efficacious but non-toxic bodily concentrations are attained.

Other drugs have also been tried as mood-regulators and include the anticonvulsants, phenytoin and sodium valproate, and cardiovascular drugs such as nifedipine, a calcium channel blocking agent. Sodium valproate is increasing in popularity.

ALTERNATIVES TO DRUG TREATMENT

Psychological therapy for bipolar disorder has not been developed or evaluated in any systematic fashion. However, many practical techniques are used and it has been shown that support group meetings, in which information both about the disorder and its treatment is given and discussed, lead to patients having a more positive attitude as well as more knowledge about the condition. In the same way, preliminary evidence suggests that treatment compliance with lithium can be improved by adding cognitive therapy.

SUMMARY

Lithium is the main line of treatment for mania and bipolar disorder. In recent years, the dosage range of lithium has been reduced, resulting in a more favourable side-effect profile but blood levels of lithium still have to be monitored routinely to avoid toxic effects. Lithium is used prophylactically to prevent attacks of mania and depression in patients with recurrent affective disorders. It may also be used to treat schizo affective disorders or added to antidepressant drugs in the treatment of patients who have not responded to one drug. In patients who do not respond to lithium, carbamazepine or antipsychotic drugs may be used. Psychological treatment for bipolar disorder has not been developed or evaluated in a systematic way as yet.

FURTHER READING

Ananth, M.D., Ghadirian, A.M. and Engelsmann, F. (1987) Lithium and memory: a review. *Canadian Journal of Psychiatry* **32**, 312–316.

Barton, C.D. Jr, Dufer, D., Monderer, R. et al. (1993) Mood variability in normal subjects on lithium. *Biological Psychiatry* **34**, 878–884.

Birch, N.J., Groft, P., Hullin, R.P. et al. (1993) Lithium prophylaxis: proposed guidelines for good clinical practice. *Lithium* **4**, 225–230.

Coryell, W., Scheftner, W., Keller, M. et al. (1993) The enduring psychosocial consequences of mania and depression. *American Journal of Psychiatry* **150**, 720–727.

Engelsmann, F., Katz, J., Ghadirian, A.M. and Schachter, D. (1988) Lithium and memory: a long-term follow-up study. *Journal of Clinical Psychopharmacology* **8**, 207–212.

Goodwin, F.K. and Jamison, K.R. (1990) *Manic-depressive Ilness*. Oxford University Press, Oxford.

Goodwin, G.M. (1994) Drug treatment in mania. *Prescribers' Journal* **34**, 19–26.

Guscott, R. and Taylor, L. (1994) Lithium prophylaxis in recurrent affective illness. Efficacy, effectiveness and efficiency. *British Journal of Psychiatry* **164**, 741–746.

Jefferson, J.W. and Greist, J.H. (1994) Lithium in psychiatry. A review. *CNS Drugs* **1**, 448–464.

Kolk, A., Kathmann, N. and Greil, W. (1993) No short-term changes of cognitive performance and mood after single doses of two different lithium retard preparations. *Pharmacopsychiatry* **26**, 235–239.

Peet, M. and Pratt, J.P. (1993) Lithium. Current status in psychiatric disorders. *Drugs* **46**, 7–17.

Shaw, E.D., Stokes, P.E., Mann, J.J. and Manevitz, A.Z.A. (1987) Effects of lithium carbonate on the memory and motor speed of bipolar outpatients. *Journal of Abnormal Psychology* **96**, 64–69.

Souza, F.G.M. and Goodwin, G.M. (1991) Lithium treatment and prophylaxis in unipolar depression: a meta-analysis. *British Journal of Psychiatry* **158**, 666–667.

Chapter 11

TREATMENT OF SCHIZOPHRENIA

The main features of schizophrenia and its treatment are discussed in this chapter. The dopamine hypothesis of schizophrenia developed from observations regarding the actions of antipsychotic drugs. These actions as well as the clinical uses and side-effects of this class of drugs are described. Increasingly, psychological management strategies are being combined with drug treatment and these are detailed.

Schizophrenia and other psychotic disorders are characterised by fundamental distortions of thinking and perception and by inappropriate or blunted affect. It is now widely accepted that the vulnerability for schizophrenia is caused by a disorder of early brain development. Both genetic and obstetric factors seem to be important. The onset may be acute, presenting with seriously disturbed behaviour or insidious with a gradual development of odd ideas and behaviour. The sufferer feels that he/she is being controlled by external forces and may lose the sense of 'self'. The features of schizophrenia can be divided into four main groups (Figure 11.1). The cognitive disturbance is shown in thought disorder of both form and content. The patient may be unable to organise his/her thoughts into a logical sequence resulting in incoherence, or speech which is very difficult to understand. Beliefs are often irrational concerning control and influence and paranoid delusions may be present. The most frequent perceptual disturbance is the presence of auditory hallucinations (hearing voices) but there may be other distortions in the quality or vividness of objects or in sensations of odour or taste. Behaviour may range from inactivity to extreme excitement and although patients often appear lacking in emotional responsiveness (flattening) they may also exhibit incongruous responses (giggling).

Schizophrenia has been classified into a number of subtypes defined by the predominant symptomatology at the time of presentation (Table 11.1). More recently a different classification system has become prevalent based on two types of schizophrenia (Table 11.2). Those patients classified as having Type 1 syndrome exhibit predominant positive symptoms and those classified as having Type 2 syndrome exhibit negative symptoms. Positive symptoms are most noticeable on initial presentation of the patient during the acute phase of

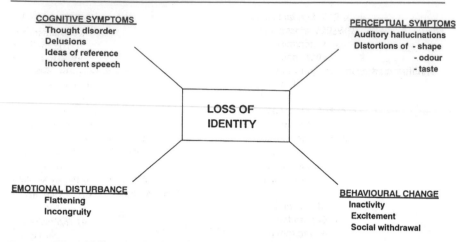

Figure 11.1   Features of schizophrenia

the disorder although they are also seen in chronic and treatment-resistant schizophrenia. Negative symptoms are more clearly seen in chronic schizophrenia. They are less responsive to drug treatment and have therefore been associated with a poor prognosis. The two types are not mutually exclusive and may occur in the same patient. In fact, factor analyses of symptom ratings have suggested three or four possible factors, the third domain representing disorganised speech and behaviour and the fourth, depression.

Table 11.1   Subtypes of schizophrenia

Subtype	Characteristics
Paranoid	Paranoid delusions Auditory hallucinations Perceptual disturbances
Disorganised Hebephrenic	Affective changes Unpredictable behaviour Mannerisms Thought disorder
Catatonic	Behavioural disturbances Negativism
Simple Residual	Blunting of affect Social withdrawal
Undifferentiated	General features

Table 11.2   Positive and negative symptoms of schizophrenia

Type 1	Positive symptoms
	Hallucinations
	Delusions
	Bizarre behaviour
	Thought disorder
	Incongruity of affect
Type 2	Negative symptoms
	Emotional flattening
	Poverty of speech/alogia
	Avolition/apathy
	Social withdrawal
	Inattention

DOPAMINE HYPOTHESIS OF SCHIZOPHRENIA

A series of observations, both clinical and behavioural-biochemical, led to the dopamine hypothesis of schizophrenia:

1. Antipsychotic drugs are efficacious in controlling the symptoms of schizophrenia. However, efficacy is limited and these drugs are also useful in the management of patients with mania, agitation and organic states.
2. Antipsychotic drugs act as antagonists at D_2 receptors, thereby lessening dopaminergic activity. However, clozapine, which has less enhanced efficacy, binds more to D_1 and 5-HT$_2$ receptors than to D_2 receptors (see p. 181).
3. Most antipsychotic drugs are fairly non-selective and block cholinergic, adrenergic, serotonergic and histaminergic receptors. Binding to these receptors does not correlate with clinical potency, whereas binding to D_2 receptors correlates highly. However, risperidone is an effective antipsychotic and yet binds much more to 5-HT$_2$ than to D_2 receptors (see p. 182).
4. Dopaminergic agonists worsen 'positive' psychotic symptoms. Such drugs include amphetamine and levodopa. However, these drugs also affect other neurotransmitter systems.

The dopamine theory of schizophrenia developed from these observations which suggested that dopaminergic mechanisms are overactive in psychosis, including schizophrenia. More direct tests of the hypothesis have been attempted, with mixed and often conflicting results. Dopamine turnover assessed by metabolite (HVA) concentrations in cerebrospinal fluid was normal in schizophrenics. Small elevations in dopamine levels in post-mortem schizophrenic brains have been reported, mainly in the nucleus accumbens and caudate nucleus. The most consistent finding has been an increase in the number of D_2 receptors in these regions of the brain. However, treatment with antipsychotic drugs increases the number of these receptors so controversy has continued as to whether this finding related to the disorder or its treatment. Results in 'drug-free' schizophrenic patients are not unanimous, one major study suggesting no abnormalities in D_2 receptors. At the very least, it is probable that relative dopaminergic overactivity underlies some aspects of psychotic behaviour such as agitation, delusions and hallucinations.

ANTIPSYCHOTIC MEDICATION

Antipsychotic drugs were an entirely novel class of therapeutic agents when they were introduced in the early 1950s. The first one, chlorpromazine, was developed in a search for new antihistamines. It was used to induce sedation and analgesia in surgical patients and was found to have a unique quietening action in first mania and then schizophrenia. However, chlorpromazine also produced movement disorders and the drugs were termed 'neuroleptics' (literally, gripping the neuron). Much later, drugs were developed which were much less likely to induce extrapyramidal effects and the term 'antipsychotic drug' was regarded as more apt.

Many antipsychotic drugs suppress vomiting and travel sickness but the main psychiatric uses are:

1. to quieten disturbed (disturbing!) patients, whatever the cause, e.g. schizophrenia, mania, brain damage,
2. to combat the symptoms of acute schizophrenia particularly delusions and hallucinations,
3. to prevent or postpone relapse of the quiescent schizophrenic patient,
4. to lessen active symptoms in the long-term schizophrenic patient,
5. in low dosage, to treat depression or anxiety in non-psychotic depressed and anxious patients (see Chapters 9 and 7 respectively).

Types of Drug

Chlorpromazine is chemically a phenothiazine and many other drugs of this class have been introduced as antipsychotics. The main subgroups are the aliphatic (chlorpromazine etc.), piperidine (thioridazine) and piperazine (trifluoperazine, fluphenazine). The first two subgroups produce many autonomic effects, but few extrapyramidal effects; the piperazine derivatives induce marked movement disorders but fewer autonomic effects. The thiothanxenes are closely related chemically to the phenothiazines and have similar subgroups. Flupenthixol and zuclopenthixol are commonly-prescribed examples. Haloperidol and related compounds are butyrophenones; pimozide is similar. The substituted benzamides (sulpiride) are another major group.

About the same time as chlorpromazine was developed, the rauwolfia alkaloids, used for centuries in Hindu traditional remedies, were introduced in the West as antihypertensive and antipsychotic drugs. Reserpine is the main active agent and exerts its pharmacological effects by depleting dopaminergic neurons of the dopamine stored at the synapse. However, reserpine was discarded in favour of the phenothiazines because its therapeutic effects were usually preceded by a phase of increased disturbance and because depressive reactions could be induced. A synthetic analogue, tetrabenazine, is still used in special indications such as Huntington's Disease.

Most preparations are available in oral and some in regular injection form for emergency use. However, in the 1960s a new type of formulation was developed for fluphenazine in which this drug was coupled to a long chain fatty acid and injected in an oily medium (depot slow-release preparation). Absorption continued over a few weeks, providing a constant level of drug cover. Many such preparations are now available.

Pharmacokinetics

Most antipsychotic drugs have complex molecular structures and their pharmacokinetics are equally complicated. Chlorpromazine, for example, has over 100 metabolites, all but a few inactive. Haloperidol has a simpler metabolic pattern.

In general, antipsychotic drugs are well-absorbed and enter the brain rapidly, sulpiride being an exception. Some, however, undergo extensive first-pass metabolism, being broken down after absorption from the gut by the liver. Depot preparations obviate this problem because they are injected into a muscle, bypassing the gut and liver.

Some relationship has been found between plasma concentrations of the antipsychotic drugs and clinical response. This is most clearly established with haloperidol. However, plasma concentrations are not routinely estimated although they may be helpful if a patient on high doses develops an adverse reaction.

Pharmacology

A series of observations led to the postulation that antipsychotic drugs (except reserpine) blocked dopamine receptors thereby inducing their therapeutic effect but also inducing extrapyramidal effects. It was suggested that dopamine mechanisms in the mesolimbic and cortical areas mediated the former effects, those in the basal ganglia the motor disorders. Other effects of dopamine blockade are to inhibit the vomiting centre in the hind-brain and to interfere with the control of growth hormones and prolactin release, thereby leading to neuroendocrine side-effects such as breast enlargement.

In humans, the affinity of various antipsychotic drugs for dopamine receptors can be estimated by measuring their displacement of compounds (ligands) selective for various types of dopamine receptor, using a neuroimaging technique such as PET or SPECT. Close correspondence is seen between D_2 receptor affinity and clinical potency, the main exceptions being clozapine and risperidone with additional affinities to D_1 and 5-HT_2 receptors, respectively. In general, about 70–90% of D_2 receptors are occupied in patients responding to antipsychotic medication and showing mild extrapyramidal effects.

Some of the acute clinical and biochemical effects of antipsychotic medication disappear with continued administration whereas others persist. Drowsiness tends to diminish after a few weeks and parkinsonism wanes within a few months. However, the elevation in prolactin levels and the clinical effects seem to persist.

Many antipsychotic drugs such as chlorpromazine have a complex pharmacology resulting from their actions on many transmitters and receptor systems. As well as their primary antipsychotic actions, secondary effects on alertness, psychomotor and cognitive functions are very obvious.

Clinical Uses

The list of indications set out earlier are a simplification of the range of uses to which these drugs are put in psychiatry. The indications often overlap or merge into each other. For example, the chronically-ill schizophrenic patient may be maintained on long-acting depot preparations but still show an increase in symptoms heralding a worsening of the condition. This pending relapse may be obviously related to some life-stress or increase in social pressures or it may appear to be spontaneous. The deteriorating situation may require an increase in dose or frequency of the depot preparation. The relapse may gather momentum so that altering the parameters of the depot preparation is too slow a manoeuvre. Oral medication may be needed or, if a severe relapse eventuates, intramuscular or even intravenous administration of an antipsychotic drug must be considered. Nevertheless, the following are the major indications.

Tranquillisation

The first psychiatric condition to be treated with chlorpromazine was actually mania but it quickly became evident to the early French investigators that disturbed behaviour of whatever aetiology responded to the drug. Chlorpromazine fairly quickly replaced the drugs previously used to quieten noisy, combative and destructive patients such as bromides, paraldehyde, barbiturates and the opiates. The drawbacks were that drowsiness could be severe, to the point of deep sleep, and bodily side-effects such as drop in blood pressure and acute dystonias (muscle spasms) might complicate the management. However, with chlorpromazine, unlike its predecessors, there was no toxic confusional psychosis to blur the clinical picture and complicate the diagnosis nor was the phase of quietening preceded by one of paradoxical excitation.

Chlorpromazine quickly became the standard treatment to tranquillise the acutely disturbed patient. Despite expressions of distaste for this 'chemical straitjacket', which have persisted to this day, it is still used. However, intramuscular injections of chlorpromazine are painful and many psychiatrists prefer to use haloperidol or droperidol intramuscularly or intravenously together with a benzodiazepine such as diazepam or lorazepam.

Acute Schizophrenia

The main line of treatment for patients suffering from acute schizophrenia is undoubtedly antipsychotic medication. Indeed, some recent studies have suggested that vigorous drug treatment should be instituted as early as possible. However, it is clear that antipsychotic medication does not cure schizophrenia but curtails the initial attack and minimises subsequent relapses. Social and employment functioning may be better maintained thereby lessening outside pressures on the patient. Despite this, perhaps up to a quarter of patients are resistant to standard antipsychotic medication and pursue a chronic or even deteriorating course. Asylum of some sort, preferably in the community, is still needed for these patients.

The effectiveness of antipsychotic medication has been supported by data from hundreds of controlled clinical trials, many involving large numbers of patients. Superiority over placebo, and over a barbiturate, is shown by greater amelioration of a wide range of symptoms, with an overall preferable side-effect profile. Symptoms which respond include belligerence, negativism, thinking disturbances, paranoid ideas, delusions and hallucinations. So-called negative symptoms such as social withdrawal and apathy (Table 11.2) do respond but much less noticeably than the positive symptoms.

No consistent differences have been found among the antipsychotic drugs with respect to efficacy (except clozapine, see p. 181). The side-effects profiles differ extensively so that the choice of medication revolves around the tolerability of various drugs to that patient. However, a patient may be encountered who responds only to one drug for obscure reasons. Sometimes, even, a response may occur to one drug at one phase of the illness and only to another later on. This unpredictability has given rise to a great deal of 'trial-and-error' medication and to the inevitable polypharmacy.

Thus, antipsychotic drugs are effective. They reduce a wide range of symptoms including fundamental ones such as thought disorder, blunted affect, withdrawal and autistic behaviour but to markedly varying extents.

Prevention of Relapse

Schizophrenia is typically a relapsing disorder with a chronic course punctuated by acute episodes of illness. Patients are usually living in the community, with relatives or friends, or in lodgings; some live in hostels with varying degrees of supervision and assistance; a few are still in the long-stay wards of psychiatric hospitals. The antipsychotic drugs suppress chronic symptoms such as hallucinations and delusions and lengthen the intervals between relapse, approximately doubling this time.

A series of studies has evaluated the efficacy of antipsychotic medication as maintenance therapy. The effectiveness differs somewhat depending on factors such as the type of patient, nature and amount of social support, home circumstances, and type of medication, particularly whether it is a depot preparation. With oral medication about 80% of those on placebo relapse over the course of a year but only a third of those maintained on phenothiazines. Those patients with previously well-integrated personalities, and affective features to their illness, seemed to benefit least from drug maintenance. Early signs of psychotic relapse include increase in delusions and hallucinations, overactivity, impaired affect and sleep disturbance. Attempts have been made to avoid long-term drug therapy but to intervene vigorously when these prodromal signs appear. Unfortunately, it is often too late then to abort the attack and most psychiatrists rely on regular maintenance medication.

The value of social work in relation to continued antipsychotic medication has been examined. The effects of social work intervention are much less than drug-placebo differences but specific counselling directed towards helping the patient adjust to his or her major role as wage-earner or homemaker is able to reduce relapse rates in patients who remain more than six months in the community. For such patients combining drugs and social worker support is the best management.

The role of relatives in influencing relapse in schizophrenic patients has been evaluated using the concept of 'expressed emotion' (EE). This is a measure derived from an interview which enumerates the critical, hostile and emotionally over-involved comments made about the patient. In patients living in a high EE environment, the relapse rate is about 50% over nine months as compared with only about 12% of those in low EE homes. The risk is greater the more time the patient spends with a high EE relative. Protection is afforded by antipsychotic medication. Patients in high EE homes, in frequent contact with an emotionally involved relative, not taking drugs, do worst.

Another factor which has been evaluated is life events. Those of an 'independent' nature, that is, outside the patient's immediate control, seem important in influencing relapse. They tend to cluster in the three weeks immediately prior to relapse and drug therapy is fairly ineffective in protecting against the influence of these events in producing relapse.

Long-acting depot preparations are better than oral medication as maintenance therapy of chronic schizophrenic patients, particularly those in the community. One factor is that the injection into the muscle avoids first-pass metabolism but the most important reason concerns compliance. Drug defaulting — failure to take medication as and when prescribed — is a general problem in all of therapeutics. But the consequences of drug defaulting in schizophrenic patients are often dramatically apparent with relapse within a few weeks. With oral medication, at least a half of patients are poor compliers. When non-trained nurses are responsible for depot injections but several care agencies are involved, the figure drops to about a third. When administrative supervision is simplified to one agency, and specialist nurses are involved, only 15% of patients default. Furthermore, with depot injections, defaulters are immediately apparent and can be followed up. Nevertheless, the prognosis even with depot injections is unsatisfactory. Even under optimal conditions, about a third of patients will relapse over two years.

Chronic Hospitalised Schizophrenics

In many Western countries, these patients constitute a diminishing band of often severely handicapped patients. Schizophrenic psychopathology may remain active and cause both symptomatic distress and behavioural problems.

Antipsychotic drugs have a limited effect on such symptoms as anxiety and restlessness. Some psychiatrists have concluded that the drugs are of little value in the management of inert, withdrawn, passive individuals, i.e. those with marked, negative symptoms. Others believe that chronic schizophrenic patients who are overactive are also not greatly helped. Studies show that patients with organic brain damage and those with dilated cerebral ventricles are particularly unresponsive.

The emphasis has shifted towards optimising the combination of social and occupational rehabilitation programmes with drug treatments. Intensive occupational therapy followed by carefully planned work schedules produces improvements which are equal or better than those of an antipsychotic drug alone. However, the best regimen is usually a combination of all available treatments — the 'total push' approach.

After withdrawal of antipsychotic medication, symptoms may worsen fairly promptly. Relapse, however, may be delayed for weeks if not months and may be related to exposure to major life events such as change of domicile or occupation. However, it is not always clear whether the life event precipitates the relapse or the relapse indirectly causes a life event to occur.

Unwanted Effects

In view of the pharmacology of the antipsychotic drugs, a wide range of side effects is inevitable (Table 11.3). Dopaminergic blockade, responsible probably for the therapeutic effects of these drugs, also accounts for some of the more important unwanted effects, in particular, the movement disorders (extrapyramidal syndromes).

Extrapyramidal Syndromes

Acute dystonia is the earliest of these neurological effects to be seen during treatment. It can even occur after a single large dose of a high-potency phenothiazine such as perphenazine. About 1 in 40 of treated patients develop this complication and it is commonest in adolescents, particularly males. The main features are often bizarre and frightening and include forced spasms of the neck (torticollis), facial grimaces, protrusion of the tongue, arching of the back (opisthotonus), sideways twisting of the trunk (scoliosis), and slurring of speech. An oculogyric crisis may occur in which the eye muscles go into spasm, usually forcing the eyes upward. Unless the attendants are aware that an antipsychotic drug has been given, the condition may be misdiagnosed as tetanus or hysteria. The condition can be relieved by the injection of an antiparkinsonian drug, which may need repeating.

Table 11.3   A comparison of the main unwanted effects of antipsychotic drugs

Drug	Unwanted effects			
	Anticholinergic effects	Sedation	Hypotension	Extrapyramidal effects
PHENOTHIAZINES				
Aliphatic				
Chlorpromazine	+ + + +	+ + + + +	+ + + + +	+ +
Piperidines				
Mesoridazine	+ + +	+ + +	+ + +	+ +
Thioridazine	+ + + + +	+ + + +	+ + + + +	+
Piperazines				
Fluphenazine	+ +	+ +	+ +	+ + + + +
Perphenazine	+ +	+ +	+ +	+ + +
Trifluoperazine	+ +	+	+ +	+ + + +
THIOXANTHENES				
Chlorprothixene	+ + + +	+ + + +	+ + + +	+ + +
Thiothixene	+ +	+ +	+ +	+ + + +
DIBENZAPINES				
Clozapine	+ + +	+ + +	+ + +	
Loxapine	+ + +	+ + +	+ +	+ + +
INDOLES				
Molindole	+ + + +	+	+ +	+ + +
BUTYROPHENONES				
Haloperidol	+	+ +	+	+ + + + +
DIPHENYLBUTYL PIPERIDINES				
Pimozide		+ +	+	+ + + + +

Akathisia ('unable to sit') is an uncontrollable urge to move, with fidgeting, squirming, standing up and sitting down repeatedly, or constant pacing up-and-down. The state is subjectively very unpleasant with intense feelings of agitation. It usually appears in the first few weeks of treatment. The condition is quite common, especially lesser degrees, and it is easy to misdiagnose it as increasing illness-related agitation. This can lead to the dose of antipsychotic drug being raised instead of lowered. Antiparkinsonian drugs are usually ineffective but a benzodiazepine or a beta-blocker may help.

The commonest of these early conditions is *parkinsonism*. The mildest form is a paucity of fine movements which can be detected by measuring the patient's handwriting (micrographia). The facial expression becomes fixed and staring. In more severe forms, the patient develops rigidity, stooped posture, small-stepping gait, coarse 'pill-rolling' tremor, excessive salivation and greasy skin (seborrhoea). Drug-induced parkinsonism is commoner in the elderly and in women. In the elderly, it may pose diagnostic problems because of its resemblance to apathy, sedation, depression or dementia. It usually comes on within a month or two of starting antipsychotic treatment but tends to wane or even disappear about six months into treatment. The incidence is directly related to the assiduity with which it is sought but up to a quarter of patients may show some of its features. A related condition is the *'rabbit'* syndrome with trembling around the mouth.

The use of antiparkinsonian medication used to be routine with the prescription of antipsychotic medication. There is no evidence that such a practice prevents parkinsonism but clear evidence of potentiation of anticholinergic effects with dry mouth, blurring of vision and constipation. The addition of a tricyclic antidepressant which may be prescribed if the schizophrenic patient becomes depressed further worsens the situation. For these reasons, it is now recommended that antiparkinsonian medication be held in reserve for when reduction of the dosage of antipsychotic medication is neither feasible nor effective. With depot injections, a few days of antiparkinsonian medication following each injection usually suffices.

The *neuroleptic malignant syndrome* comprises catatonia, akinesia (lack of movement), twitching (chorea), difficulty in swallowing, speaking and breathing. Rise in temperature may be life-threatening. This not uncommon condition usually follows a brisk rise in dosage of a high-potency antipsychotic such as haloperidol. The antipsychotic drug must be withdrawn and supportive measures instituted.

Tardive dyskinesia (TD) is a syndrome which comes on after months or years of antipsychotic drug treatment (tardive = belated) and is characterised by abnormal, coordinated, stereotyped involuntary movements (dyskinesia). These fluctuate in severity and disappear during sleep. Some patients have major and crippling dyskinesias but most suffer only minor effects. The prevalence is quite high with up to 40% of long-term users showing the condition, almost all with minor severity. It is not usually progressive.

The muscles of the face, especially around the mouth and the tongue, are the most commonly affected. Often the tongue or the floor of the mouth quivers; this may be the earliest or the only sign. More serious forms of TD involve the limb muscles or those of the back or of respiration. Complications include ulceration of the mouth, extrusion of food while chewing, impaired swallowing and difficulty with walking.

The condition may involve more fixed spasms of muscles rather than repetitive movements; it is then termed 'tardive dystonia'.

TD or tardive dystonia may occur for the first time when antipsychotic drugs are discontinued. Re-institution of antipsychotic medication may suppress the TD but this tends to be temporary.

Age is an important factor predisposing to TD. Indeed, some aged normal individuals show mild TD-like movements despite never being exposed to an antipsychotic drug. Older patients are more likely to develop an irreversible form; in younger patients, the condition often reverses after stopping treatment. Although antipsychotic drugs are usually involved, other drugs acting on dopamine mechanisms have occasionally been implicated.

The basis of TD is unclear and no simple mechanism can explain the delay in its appearance. The consensus is that dopaminergic pathways are distorted in some complex way but that other neurotransmitters such as GABA and 5-HT may also be involved.

The treatment of TD is largely unsatisfactory, at least beyond the short-term. Increasing the dose of antipsychotic medication or substituting a more potent one may help for a while, as noted above. Similarly, giving a dopamine-depleting drug like tetrabenazine provides only a temporary expedient. Benzodiazepines and drugs acting directly on GABA systems such as sodium valproate have some beneficial effects but this may be mainly non-specific sedative actions. The general strategy is to minimise the dosage of anti-psychotic drug, avoid antiparkinsonian medication, and to use benzodiazepines as judiciously as possible, intermittent use being the safest. Prevention is an important goal, reserving antipsychotic medication for those with unequivocal signs of psychosis and the definite diagnosis of schizophrenia.

Autonomic Effects

Some of the antipsychotic drugs such as thioridazine and chlorpromazine have marked anticholinergic effects and produce dry mouth, blurred vision and constipation. The other antipsychotic drugs such as trifluoperazine, haloperidol and sulpiride are much less potent in this respect. More serious untoward effects include retention of urine and paralysis of bowel function and are much more likely when other drugs with anticholinergic properties are co-prescribed.

Antipsychotic drugs also have alpha-adrenergic blocking effects and this can result in a major drop in blood pressure on standing up; the patient may feel dizzy or faint.

Endocrine Effects

Prolactin is a hormone involved in the regulation of milk production but is also present in non-lactating women and in men. Its production is inhibited by dopamine. Antipsychotic drugs, by blocking dopamine, release this inhibition and prolactin levels increase. This can result in the spurious production of milk and suppression of menstrual periods in women, and in loss of libido in men.

Weight gain is often very marked because of disturbances of appetite, possibly related to blockade of serotonin pathways. Several kilos can accrue within a few years, and may distress the patient. Dietary control is the only feasible measure.

Neuroleptic-induced Deficit Syndrome

Another adverse effect, the source of some controversy, is the possible induction of depression. However, schizophrenic patients may present initially with marked depressive symptoms and suicide is 50 times more frequent in such patients than in the general population. Each episode of the illness may develop into a depressive phase before resolving. The role of antipsychotic drug therapy is therefore difficult to clarify. A further complication is that some but not all antipsychotic drugs have definite mood-elevating properties. Use of a drug without this secondary effect may by contrast appear 'depressiogenic'.

The subjective 'load' imposed on the schizophrenic patient has been an increasing source of concern especially as attempts are made to treat more and more of these patients in the community. The advent of newer antipsychotic drugs with fewer subjective effects has focused attention on the cognitive, psychomotor and motivational deficits suffered by the patient. How much is illness-related — negative symptoms etc? How much is related to depression? And how much reflects the effects of the drugs on mood, motivation and cognitive functioning. The term 'neuroleptic-induced deficit syndrome' has recently been coined to cover these possible effects of antipsychotic drugs.

Adverse Effects and Overdose

The antipsychotic drugs are associated with a long list of uncommon but nevertheless significant adverse effects. These include jaundice, drop in white blood count, pigmentation of skin and eye and changes in the electro-cardiogram. High doses may be associated with sudden, unexpected death.

The antipsychotic drugs are frequently used in overdose, both deliberate and accidental. The toxicity is lower than that of the tricyclic antidepressants but death can occur with respiratory depression, cardiac irregularities or epileptic fits. Treatment is supportive and symptomatic, no specific antidote being available.

SOME NEWER ANTIPSYCHOTIC DRUGS

Clozapine

Clozapine is the only antipsychotic drug licensed for the treatment of schizo-phrenic patients resistant to other antipsychotic drugs. This reflects both its enhanced efficacy and its serious untoward effects. It has a broad spectrum of pharmacological properties but has an atypical profile. Thus, it is a weak antagonist of D_2 receptors but also blocks D_1 (and D_4) receptors. Clozapine also acts as an antagonist at 5-HT_2, alpha$_1$ and alpha$_2$-adrenergic, histaminic (H_1) and acetylcholine (muscarinic receptors). In animals, it blocks D_1 more than D_2 receptors, a finding replicated in schizophrenic patients using neuroimaging techniques. The drug does not induce supersensitivity in dopamine systems subserving movement functions and it raises plasma prolactin levels only ephemerally. It may act preferentially on mesolimbic (emotional) rather than striatal (movement) mechanisms. The biochemical basis for its unique profile remains elusive.

Clozapine is well-absorbed, with large inter-patient variations in plasma concentrations and rate of metabolism. It has a half-life ranging from 6–26 hours.

The drug has been studied for over 30 years. In the early 1970s, its efficacy in schizophrenia was established in acute schizophrenic patients, 60–80% of whom responded in a few weeks. However, a spate of adverse effects occurred, the drug lowering the white blood count to levels incompatible with defence against infections (agranulocytosis). Consequently, several patients died and the drug, although left available in some countries, was withdrawn by the manufacturers from worldwide development. Several clinicians overcame the reluctance of the pharmaceutical company to evaluate clozapine. They showed that 30–60% of patients who had failed to respond to several previous trials of medication did well with clozapine over six weeks to six months of observation. The risk of agranulocytosis was minimised by regular, usually weekly, monitoring of the white blood cell count. The main study involved 319 schizophrenic patients who had already failed to respond to at least three courses of treatment. They were treated prospectively with haloperidol but fewer than 2% improved: 268 of the non-responders were treated with either chlorpromazine or clozapine. Very clear superiority for clozapine was demonstrated both for positive and negative symptoms.

About 3% of patients treated with clozapine show a significant drop in white blood cells but only in very few does it drop to dangerously inadequate levels. Cessation of clozapine is almost invariably followed by recovery of the bone-marrow. A rigorous patient monitoring service is in place in most countries where it is used extensively. Thus, clozapine is deemed to have a favourable risk/benefit ratio in severely ill schizophrenic patients but not otherwise.

The most common adverse effects of clozapine are sedation, excessive salivation, dizziness, constipation, weight gain and drop in blood-pressure. Up to 3 or 4% of patients on clozapine develop epileptic fits but this can usually be obviated by modest dosage. On the bonus side, clozapine is less likely to induce movement disorders than typical antipsychotics, and TD is rare in patients taking clozapine alone. Rebound psychosis may follow discontinuation of clozapine and may lead on to difficulties stabilising patients on other drugs.

Risperidone

This new drug binds strongly to $5\text{-}HT_2$ receptors and less avidly to D_2 receptors. It also acts as an antagonist at $alpha_1$ and H_1 receptors. In animal preparations it blocks the actions of both serotonin and dopamine. Risperidone has a long duration of action. Clinical data are so far limited but the drug seems to have at least the antipsychotic potency of typical antipsychotic drugs with a lower incidence of extrapyramidal effects. Like older drugs, however, it can cause low blood pressure and endocrine disturbances.

Psychological Effects

The effects of antipsychotic drugs in schizophrenic patients are much less marked than in healthy controls. Schizophrenic patients have pronounced performance deficits before treatment and many attempts have been made to investigate these. The following can only be a brief summary of this work.

Cognitive Deficits in Schizophrenia

The performance of patients with schizophrenia is not only inferior to that of healthy controls but also to that of controls with other psychiatric illnesses on almost any difficult or demanding task. In fact a disturbance of cognition is considered a cardinal feature of the disorder. This generalised disability is probably related to very basic neural dysfunction occurring developmentally. There is no evidence of a progressive decline during the adult life of schizophrenics which is distinct from other dementing disorders. However, this broad deficit does not obviate more specific, localised dysfunctions in individual patients or with particular syndromes. Schizophrenia is a heterogeneous disorder and attempts have been made to relate areas of symptomatology to specific cognitive deficits. Thus, it has been proposed that the two or three main symptom clusters relate to specific neuropsychological deficits. Overall, attempts to correlate syndromes with specific deficits have not been particularly successful. This is probably because task performance may be impaired to the same extent by both negative and positive symptoms but the way in which it is impaired may be different. An explanatory framework is necessary to predict results. In one such framework it has been proposed that the central impairment in schizophrenia is in the initiation and monitoring of actions. There are two routes to action, one dependent on external factors and one driven by internal goals and willed intentions. Schizophrenics with negative symptoms should have difficulty generating action based on internal goals. Those with positive symptoms should have difficulty monitoring and correcting errors. Research using this model has found some results compatible with the predictions for negative symptoms but as low motivation is a prime negative symptom this may be confounding the results. There is also evidence of a significant variability in symptoms over time which indicates a difficulty in associating time-limited states of phenomenology with fundamental neuropsychological deficits.

Information processing abnormalities with reference to high processing loads have been found not just in actively psychotic patients but also in remitted and schizotypal patients and may reflect vulnerability factors for a schizophrenic disorder. These attentional deficits may be related to a reduction in available processing capacity for task relevant cognitive operations. There are many possible causative factors but there is evidence that this difficulty in processing information is due to an inability to inhibit irrelevant information from gaining attentional resources (distractibility). This has been termed the defective filter theory but has been challenged by those who believe that the schizophrenic's difficulty in organising and maintaining an effective strategy for processing information is related to response set rather than a filtering defect. This formulation suggests that schizophrenics are less able to make use of the redundancy and patterning of sensory input. Actively psychotic or chronic patients continue to display impairment even when demands on processing capacity are low and this may reflect a more severe and pervasive information processing deficit. Overall intellectual impairment is a result of bilateral CNS dysfunction but attempts have been made to relate more specific neuropsychological deficits to frontal and temporal regions. Debate continues as to whether cognitive deficits are lateralised in origin although most authors favour a left-hemisphere interpretation.

Cognitive inflexibility due to a dysfunction in the frontal lobes has been inferred from poor performance on the Wisconsin Card Sorting Test (WCST). An inordinate number of studies has used this task and found an increase in perseverative errors in various groups of schizophrenics. However, a cautionary note to the interpretation of a permanent or irreversible deficit has been given by results showing monetary reinforcement can decrease errors. It seems that reward for correct performance can enable patients to inhibit irrelevant information and direct attentional resources to the task-relevant features. Practice on task has also been shown to improve performance. Recently regional cerebral blood flow measures taken during WCST performance which have been coregistered with magnetic resonance imaging have also implicated a dysfunction of a prefrontal-limbic network in schizophrenia.

Evidence has also accrued for dysfunction in the medial temporal lobes. Deficits in long-term and semantic memory which are disproportionate to the general level of intellectual impairment have been found. Learning and memory performance has been assessed in monozygotic twins discordant for schizophrenia. Affected twins show impairment on most tasks indicating diffuse cortical dysfunction but deficits are most severe on tests of vigilance, memory and concept formation suggesting that dysfunction is greatest in the frontotemporal cortex. A clinical measure of global level of functioning is strongly associated with level of cognitive performance but manifest symptoms are not highly associated with neuropsychological scores.

Several studies have shown that schizophrenics find it difficult to generate ideas or organise information spontaneously without the help of external stimuli. In word fluency tasks, this has been shown to be a consequence of deficiencies in the retrieval process. Both poverty of speech (a negative feature) and incoherence of speech (a positive feature) reflect problems with retrieval of words from the lexicon. A reduced ability to generate words is more marked in patients with negative features whereas those with positive features are more likely to produce inappropriate words. However, a similar degree of memory impairment is found in association with both negative symptoms and formal thought disorder. Interestingly, performance can be improved by encouragement and direction. It seems likely that schizophrenics perform poorly on standardised neuropsychological tests partly because they have been validated on normals with standardised instructions. Schizo-phrenics might benefit from fuller instructions and testing in a positive non-threatening environment. However, it is likely that deficits in high-level problem solving will remain.

Effects of Antipsychotics in Healthy Volunteers

The side-effects of anti-psychotic drugs are much greater in healthy volunteers and so in most studies very low doses have been administered to ascertain psychological effects. Sedative compounds such as chlorpromazine tend to produce extreme tiredness. Subjects report this as unpleasant and accompanied by slower, confused thinking, difficulty in concentrating and feeling clumsy. Clozapine induces a desire to sleep. Less sedative compounds like perphenazine, trifluoperazine and haloperidol induce dysphoria and restlessness. In one study in which antipsychotic doses of haloperidol were administered to healthy controls, the subjects were found to be two to four times more likely than patients to experience dystonias, restlessness and sedation and thus to require anticholinergic medication.

The effects of antipsychotics on performance in healthy subjects are related to their sedative properties and to dose. Doses of chlorpromazine causing sedation also produce non-specific widespread impairment of performance. In lower doses the effects are more pronounced on tests of sustained attention than on brief cognitive tasks (DSST). Some studies have missed potential impairment by testing too soon after intake. Maximal effects occur two to four hours later.

There have been far fewer studies of other antipsychotics but little impairment has been shown after either perphenazine or trifluoperazine. The effects of haloperidol are related to dose and testing time. Little impairment has been found before four hours but impairment on tasks of attention and rapid information processing has been found after 4–6 hours. Droperidol, given IV, caused some decreases in attention capacity and processing speed but there was a suggestion that it might facilitate attentional shift. Flupenthixol (given orally) has been shown to produce some detrimental effects on perceptual and psychomotor functioning but only after repeated doses (four days).

Newer atypical compounds produce dissimilar effects. Sulpiride has not been shown to cause any impairment after either single or repeated doses. Clozapine like chlorpromazine is very sedative and in one study has produced impairment on both psychomotor and cognitive tasks.

Low doses of conventional antipsychotic drugs can therefore cause impairment on a range of tasks but this is most noticeable on tasks of sustained attention or rapid information processing rather than higher cognitive functions. Non-sedative compounds like trifluoperazine and sulpiride produce no discernible impairment.

Effects of Antipsychotics in Schizophrenic Patients

Although antipsychotics, and sedative compounds in particular, produce impairment on sustained attention and some psychomotor tasks in healthy volunteers, much larger doses produce minimal effects in schizophrenic patients taking such medication chronically. Acute administration can impair some aspects of performance but this generally resolves with chronic treatment. Unfortunately many of the studies have not controlled factors such as severity of psychopathology and randomisation to treatment let alone pharmacological factors such as washout periods, other drug use, etc. and there are few studies directly comparing different compounds.

Studies examining the acute administration of antipsychotic drugs to schizophrenic patients have found some impairment on sustained attention, coding and manual dexterity. However these effects not only diminish over time but are converted to improvement after several weeks treatment. After eight weeks' treatment with an optimal dose (excessive doses may again show impairments) improved performance has been shown on a number of neuropsychological tasks — sustained attention, visuospatial ability, word association — but no change has been found on measures of abstract thinking, problem solving or memory function. It may be that no improvement has been found on these higher cognitive functions because of the anticholinergic properties of some standard antipsychotic drugs or the concomitant use of anticholinergic medication to treat extrapyramidal side effects. Nevertheless patients treated with antipsychotics are more amenable to neurocognitive rehabilitation (programmes designed to improve psychological functioning) and those treated with less sedative and less anticholinergic compounds may do better. Generally speaking, psychological improvement parallels clinical recovery and may continue to improve for several months. Therefore the treatment benefits of antipsychotic drugs far outweigh any subtle impairment of performance after acute doses.

It is important that future studies match patients for initial severity and symptom clusters in order that potential cognitive improvements are discernible.

SOME ASPECTS OF MANAGEMENT

A patient suffering a schizophrenic breakdown may become acutely ill and require intensive treatment which usually includes large doses of tranquillising drugs. A typical regimen for the very disturbed, hostile, combative, agitated patient is haloperidol 10 mg and diazepam 10 mg both given intravenously. About two-thirds of patients quieten down after this but the remainder will need a repeat injection. The experience of the nursing staff is crucial in managing such psychotic individuals. In addition, heavy sedation needs careful monitoring to avoid undue stress on the heart or respiratory depression.

Most patients suffer a more gradual relapse or do not develop acutely disturbed phases needing emergency medication. Instead, the patient becomes more anxious, panicky or depressed, or his/her psychotic symptoms such as hallucinations and delusions intensify. Withdrawal, irritability, suspicion, perplexity and preoccupation with odd ideas often supervene. Although some patients may need admission to hospital, most can be managed successfully at home. Indeed, a hospital admission may represent a major setback to the patient not only symptomatically but in terms of social and occupational functioning. The anxiety of both patient and carers may quickly subside as medical and social services are mobilised. Drug dosage may need increasing or more careful supervision insisted on if the patient is suspected of poor compliance. Zuclopenthixol acetate (Clopixol Acuphase) acts for up to 72 hours and can be given by intramuscular injection if the patient's level of disturbance is increasing at a rapid rate.

Nevertheless, hospital admission may be inevitable if the patient is non-compliant, lacks support, is self-neglectful or violent. Admission under an appropriate section of the Mental Health Act may be needed.

About 25% of people with schizophrenic breakdowns make a good recovery. At the other extreme 1 in 10 do badly, become mentally disabled and need long-term residential care. Increasingly, such care is being provided in the community instead of the old-style asylums, but some fall through the net and end up homeless.

The middle two-thirds of the severity spectrum is occupied by patients with some persisting symptoms, social problems and relapses. Patients with so-called negative symptoms of withdrawal, apathy, neglect, flatness of emotion and lack of motivation tend to do poorly. Antipsychotic drugs given as maintenance therapy are the mainstay of management and this about doubles the interval between relapses. Careful monitoring of therapy is essential and most care teams try to minimise the medication because of unpleasant side effects such as sedation and movement disorders. Compliance is often poor and depot injection treatment is often essential to keep the patient functioning.

Acute relapses are often associated with major life events such as change of job or bereavement. Extra careful monitoring is necessary at these times. The relapse rate may be reduced by altering the social environment of the patient to make it less stressful. One aspect of this is to work with the family to lower its level of 'expressed emotion', to change critical involvement to tolerant support. Although many families successfully effect this change, a few are resistant to even acknowledging that one of their members is mentally ill.

Maintenance of the patient is a tight-rope between overstimulation — stressful criticism and urging of the patient beyond their capabilities — and understimulation — the benign neglect of the old mental hospitals. A careful, flexible plan for rehabilitation is essential with a structured work and personal environment which increases in complexity at a governable pace. Accommodation moves from the hospital to high-dependency hostels and on to a semi-independent existence in a group home and then a flat-share, culminating in independence. Employment ranges from occupational therapy to day centres, rehabilitation workshops, industrial centres, and the open labour market.

The emphasis of care has shifted to community mental health teams (CMHT). Each patient is allocated a key worker or case manager, typically a community psychiatric nurse or a social worker. The key worker is closely involved with the family or hostel staff; the case manager is usually more supervisory. Increasingly, general practitioners are becoming involved in the active management of major psychiatric disorders, and are especially helpful supporting the carers. They often know the whole family, have seen the initial episodes and can provide care for any physical problems suffered by the patient. Coordination between CMHTs and GPs is essential to maintain good clinical care. Domiciliary visits may be needed, especially if problems arise, and psychiatric help may then be appropriate. Voluntary agencies may also be involved, and are invaluable in educating and supporting the family. In particular, they can assuage the self-guilt which many families feel, especially when someone has misguidedly implied that they are chiefly responsible for inducing the patient's illness. Discussing problems with other similarly-placed families provides invaluable support.

COMBINATION OF ANTIPSYCHOTIC DRUGS WITH PSYCHOLOGICAL MANAGEMENT STRATEGIES

Although antipsychotic drugs are the mainstay of treatment for sufferers of schizophrenia, many patients continue to experience residual psychotic symptoms and some are refractory to standard antipsychotics. This has led to the re-emergence of clozapine and the experimentation with other $5\text{-}HT_2$ receptor antagonists among drug treatment and to a search for additional or alternative psychological ways to manage persistent symptoms. These approaches have followed four broad pathways (Table 11.4). Psychological approaches have generally been implemented in addition to drugs. No

Table 11.4 Psychological approaches to the management of schizophrenia

Family intervention
Neurocognitive rehabilitation
Behavioural techniques
Cognitive therapy

controlled trials have compared psychological treatment with drugs but in well-designed studies, medication has been kept stable while the addition of a specific treatment has been compared with standard psychiatric care. One meta-analysis of over 100 trials comparing various treatments found that social intervention, but not psychotherapy, enhanced the effects of standard drug treatment.

Family Intervention

This work originated from research on expressed emotion. There are many reviews on the topic but a recent one which looked at 25 studies, showed a twofold difference in relapse rates over nine months for schizophrenia between low (median rate = 21%) and high (48%) EE families. Although research has shown that high EE relatives tend to exhibit negatively charged behaviours which are then reciprocated by patients it is not known which factors initiate or terminate these interactions. High EE in families is influenced by numerous factors including socio-economic status, the burden experienced by relatives in terms of length and severity of the patient's illness, their understanding of the illness, their methods of coping with it and the availability and use of social support agencies. It has been found that caretakers of chronic schizophrenic patients are twice as likely to suffer from psychological ill health as the general population but little is known of the effectiveness of differential ways of coping. Relatives with more contact with professionals report higher satisfaction and there have been a number of family intervention studies aimed both at reducing high levels of EE and the overall burden. Four family-therapy models have been developed (Table 11.5). While all have shown some efficacy, the studies have concentrated on high EE families and have neglected low EE families who may have a high degree of social impairment. Only behavioural family management has also been evaluated by an independent group of researchers in low EE families. It is able to reduce relapse rates at one year from 55% to 14% and is beneficial for patients from both high and low EE homes. Brief intervention studies offer only 2–10 sessions of education. These generally improve relatives' knowledge of the illness and alleviate some of the burden but the

Table 11.5 Family therapy models

Behavioural family management	— Falloon et al. (1984)
Social intervention	— Leff et al. (1985)
Community management	— Tarrier et al. (1989)
Family psychoeducation	— Hogarty et al. (1991)

involvement only of relatives with the exclusion of patients means no effects are found on patient functioning. Other studies have focused on the attitudes of patients and relatives rather than EE. Patients with frequent contact with a relative they view as positive have less chance of psychotic exacerbation and patients whose expectations of their parents are not fulfilled have the most negative outcome.

Neurocognitive Rehabilitation

The nature of the schizophrenic illness produces profound effects on psychological functioning seen both on formal testing and in everyday living. The integrated psychological therapy (IPT) programme was developed to specifically redress these deficiencies. It comprises 5 subprogrammes (Table 11.6) designed to ameliorate both cognitive dysfunctions and social behavioural deficits. IPT has been evaluated in several independent studies and has shown favourable overall effects both on cognitive and psychopathological measures. There is however little evidence demonstrating the generalisability of these improvements. It has generally been administered as group training but a preliminary report of a modified programme based on putative prefrontal/frontal executive functions and administered intensively over eight weeks on an individual basis has claimed not only improvement in lower order cognitive functions and daily living skills but also clearer thinking and improved functioning. It is likely that future cognitive remediation programmes will gain from cognitive psychology as well as neuropsychology and will target attention, memory and executive functioning but it is

Table 11.6 Integrated psychological therapy

Interpersonal problem solving
Social skills
Verbal communication
Social perception
Cognitive differentiation

important that the issue of generalisability of training to outside the immediate target functions is addressed.

Behavioural Techniques

Behaviour modification techniques based on the principles of operant conditioning were investigated in the 1950s and 1960s. The approach was known as 'token economy'. Tokens were used to reward chronic, institutionalised patients when they behaved appropriately. Tokens could be exchanged for privileges on the ward. Such schemes are still devised by psychologists for individual patients in such settings and have been shown to augment response over standard drug treatment. Behavioural techniques such as social skills training are often used as part of a management or family intervention strategy and communication skills can be taught in an educational or rehabilitation package. These have been aimed at negative symptoms or poor social functioning. However, it is apparent that patients also use behavioural techniques to combat positive symptoms such as hallucinations and delusions. They report using distraction, ignoring, selective listening and setting limits and In one case audiotape therapy.

Cognitive Therapy

Cognitive behavioural techniques have also been used in schizophrenia. Patients have been trained in procedures such as problem-solving to help them to identify and tackle interpersonal difficulties. Very recently a controlled trial (the first of its kind) compared two alternative cognitive-behavioural methods: coping strategy enhancement (CSE) and problem solving (PS) (Tarrier et al., 1993). The first (CSE) attempts to identify already existing coping strategies and reinforce these by training the patient to cope with and control both the cues and reactions to symptoms and the second (PS) attempts to teach a cognitive plan for problem solving and to encourage its application. Treatment was given in 10 sessions over five weeks. The difficulties implicit in such a study are evident from the fact that of 48 suitable patients and 39 actually recruited, only 27 completed treatment but the results were encouraging for both treatments. Patients showed a significant improvement on target symptoms but this did not generalise to wider areas of social or cognitive functioning.

Cognitive techniques have also been used to modify delusional beliefs. Beliefs about the power, identity and purpose of their voices (auditory hallucinations) have been shown to underlie people's behaviour towards them. Cognitive therapy sets out to elucidate and challenge these core beliefs. Because such beliefs vary with clinical state, it is important to have adequate baseline data, independent ratings and follow-up assessments after treatment termination but few studies have met these criteria. However, methodologically strong studies have shown impressive results in single case designs. The techniques used to dispute beliefs comprised hypothetical contradiction and structured verbal challenge followed by testing the beliefs empirically (reality-testing intervention). Not only did this approach lead to reductions in belief conviction and concomitant distress but this improvement was associated with a reduction in voice activity and increased adaptive behaviour. If such results can be confirmed in larger controlled studies, then they will have far-reaching consequences.

Cognitive-behavioural techniques have therefore been shown to improve symptoms refractory to drug treatment but it is too early to say whether such effects are limited to the areas targeted or may be generalisable. It may be that different approaches are helpful with different symptoms or that more intensive or longer treatment periods are required.

SUMMARY

Schizophrenia is the most severe psychiatric disorder which is frequently associated with severe morbidity. It is widely believed to be caused by a disorder of early brain development. The advent of antipsychotic drug treatment has made a major contribution to the management of schizophrenia, allowing patients to live and be treated in the community. Antipsychotic drugs are not only used to quieten disturbed behaviour and control symptoms in acute schizophrenia but also to prevent or postpone relapse in the chronic disorder. It is thought that antipsychotics exert their therapeutic effects by blocking dopamine receptors but this also induces extrapyramidal symptoms. Newer drugs with different pharmacological profiles have a lower incidence of EPS. Schizophrenia is associated with a widespread but nonprogressive deterioration in cognitive function. High level problem-solving deficits are not improved by drug treatment and are likely to impair both work performance and social relationships. Psychological strategies have been developed to improve functioning and alleviate these difficulties.

FURTHER READING

Bollini, P., Pampallona, S., Orza, M.J., Adams, M.E. and Chalmers, T.C. (1994) Antipsychotic drugs: is more worse? A meta-analysis of the published randomized control trials. *Psychological Medicine* **24**, 307–316.

Braff, D.L. (1991) Information processing and attentional abnormalities in schizophrenic disorders. In *Cognitive Bases of Mental Disorders* (Magaro, P.A., ed.). Sage Publications, Newbury Park, CA, pp. 262–307.

Brenner, H.D., Hodel, B., Roder, V. and Corrigan, P. (1992) Treatment of cognitive dysfunctions and behavioral deficits in schizophrenia: integrated psychological therapy. *Schizophrenia Bulletin* 18, 21–26.

Cassens, G., Inglis, A.K., Appelbaum, P.S. and Gutheil, T.G. (1990) Neuroleptics: effects on neuropsychological function in chronic schizophrenic patients. *Schizophrenia Bulletin* 16, 477–499.

Coffey, I. (1994) Options for the treatment of negative symptoms of schizophrenia. *CNS Drugs* 1, 107–118.

Corcoran, R. and Frith, C.D. (1993) Neuropsychology and neurophysiology in schizophrenia. *Current Opinion in Psychiatry* 6, 74–79.

Davies, L.M. and Drummond, M.F. (1993) Assessment of costs and benefits of drug therapy for treatment-resistant schizophrenia in the United Kingdom. *British Journal of Psychiatry* 162, 38–42.

Davis, J.M., Metalon, L., Watanabe, M.D. and Blake, L. (1994) Depot antipsychotic drugs. Place in therapy. *Drugs* 47, 741–773.

Falloon, I., Boyd, J. and McGill, C. (1984) *Family Care of Schizophrenia: A Problem-Solving Approach to the Treatment of Mental Illness.* Guilford Press, New York.

Frith, C.D. (1992) *The Cognitive Neuropsychology of Schizophrenia.* Lawrence Erlbaum Associates, Hillsdale, USA and Hove, UK.

Goldberg, T.E., Greenberg, R.D., Griffin, S.J. et al. (1993) The effect of clozapine on cognition and psychiatric symptoms in patients with schizophrenia. *British Journal of Psychiatry* 162, 43–48.

Goldberg, T.E., Torrey, E.F., Gold, J.M., Ragland, J.D., Bigelow, L.B. and Weinberger, D.R. (1993) Learning and memory in monozygotic twins discordant for schizophrenia. *Psychological Medicine* 23, 71–85.

Grant, S. and Fitton, A. (1994) Risperidone. A review of its pharmacology and therapeutic potential in the treatment of schizophrenia. *Drugs* 48, 253–273.

Green, M.F. Cognitive remediation in schizophrenia: Is it time yet? *American Journal of Psychiatry* 150, 178–187.

Häfner, H., Gattaz, W.F. and Janzarik W. (eds) (1987) *Search for the Causes of Schizophrenia.* Springer-Verlag, Berlin.

Heaton, R., Paulsen, J.S., McAdams, L.A. et al. (1994) Neuropsychological deficits in schizophrenics. Relationship to age, chronicity, and dementia. *Archives of General Psychiatry* 51, 469–476.

Hogarty, G., Anderson, M., Reiss, D. et al. (1991) Family psychoeducation, social skills training and maintenance chemotherapy in the aftercare treatment of schizophrenia: II. Two-year effects of a controlled study on relapse and adjustment. *Archives of General Psychiatry* 48, 340–347.

Kane, J.M. (1993) Newer antipsychotic drugs. *Drugs* 46, 585–593.

Kavanagh, D.J. (1992) Recent developments in expressed emotion and schizophrenia. *British Journal of Psychiatry* 160, 601–620.

King, D.J. (1990) The effect of neuroleptics on cognitive and psychomotor function. *British Journal of Psychiatry* 157, 799–811.

Kingdon, D.G. and Turkington, D. (1994) *Cognitive-Behavioral Therapy of Schizophrenia.* Guilford Press, New York.

Lam, D.H. (1991) Psychosocial family intervention in schizophrenia: A review of empirical studies. *Psychological Medicine* 21, 423–441.

Leff, J., Kuipers, L., Berkowitz, R. and Sturgeon, D. (1985) A controlled trial of social intervention in families of schizophrenic patients: two-year follow-up. *British Journal of Psychiatry* **146**, 594–600.

Lowe, C.F. and Chadwick, P.D.J. (1990) Verbal control of delusions. *Behavior Therapy* **21**, 461–479.

Miller, A.L., Maas, J.W., Contreras, S. et al. (1993) Acute effects of neuroleptics on unmedicated schizophrenic patients and controls. *Biological Psychiatry* **34**, 178–187.

Morice, R.D. and Delahunty, A. (1993) Treatment strategies for the remediation of neurocognitive dysfunction in schizophrenia. In *The Neuropsychology of Schizophrenia* (Pantelis, C., Nelson, H.E. and Barnes, T., eds). Wiley, Chichester.

Nuechterlein, K.H., Dawson, M.E., Gitlin, M., Snyder, K.S., Yee, C.M. and Mintz, J. (1992) Developmental processes in schizophrenic disorders: longitudinal studies of vulnerability and stress. *Schizophrenia Bulletin* **18**, 387–425.

Nyberg, S., Farde, L., Eriksson, L., Halldin, C. and Eriksson, B. (1993) 5-HT$_2$ and D$_2$ dopamine receptor occupancy in the living human brain. *Psychopharmacology* **110**, 265–272.

Randolph, E.T., Eth, S., Glynn, S.M. et al. (1994) Behavioural family management in schizophrenia. Outcome of a clinic-based intervention. *British Journal of Psychiatry* **164**, 501–506.

Romme, M.A.J., Honig, A., Noorthoorn, E.O. and Escher, A.D.M.A.C. (1992) Coping with hearing voices: an emancipatory approach. *British Journal of Psychiatry* **161**, 99–103.

Saykin, A.J., Shtasel, D.L., Gur, R.E. et al. (1994) Neuropsychological deficits in neuroleptic naive patients with first-episode schizophrenia. *Archives of General Psychiatry* **51**, 124–131.

Summerfelt, A.T., Alphs, L.D., Wagman, A.M.I., Funderburk, F.R., Hierholzer, R.M. and Strauss, M.E. (1991) Reduction of perseverative errors in patients with schizophrenia using monetary feedback. *Journal of Abnormal Psychology* **100**, 613–616.

Tarrier, N., Barrowclough, C., Vaughn, C. et al. (1989) Community management of schizophrenia: a two-year follow-up of a behavioural intervention with families. *British Journal of Psychiatry* **154**, 625–628.

Tarrier, N., Beckett, R., Harwood, S., Baker, A., Yusupoff, L. and Ugarteburu, I. (1993) A trial of two cognitive-behavioural methods of treating drug-resistant residual psychotic symptoms in schizophrenic patients: I. Outcome. *British Journal of Psychiatry* **162**, 524–532.

Weinberger, D.R., Berman, K.F., Suddath, R. and Torrey, E.F. (1992) Evidence of a dysfunction of a prefrontal-limbic network in schizophrenia: a magnetic resonance imaging and regional cerebral blood flow study of discordant monozygotic twins. *American Journal of Psychiatry* **149**, 890–897.

Windgassen, K. (1992) Treatment with neuroleptics: the patient's perspective. *Acta Psychiatrica Scandinavica* **86**, 405–410.

Chapter 12

DRUG TREATMENT OF ALCOHOL AND DRUG DEPENDENCE

This chapter is not intended as a review of the problems of drugs of addiction, i.e. those abused or misused in a non-medical context. Rather it is an outline of the clinical pharmacology of the drugs which are used to treat people with drug problems, either to facilitate withdrawal and detoxification or to promote moderation or abstinence. The principles of action and mode of usage provide some useful illustrations of the complexity of psychotropic drug interactions and also of drug and non-drug interventions and their relationship in clinical practice. In view of the increasing prevalence of alcohol- and drug-related problems, the health-care professional is more and more likely to encounter people presenting practical difficulties.

ALCOHOL-RELATED PROBLEMS

Alcohol is the most commonly abused drug and provides an example of complicated social, personal and pharmacological interactions. Most people are in complete control of their drinking, some lose control on rare occasions and yet others are regularly in thrall to their habit and may be physically dependent. Although the extent of alcohol-related problems broadly parallels inversely the real cost of alcohol, individual and even genetic factors are important. Despite the chemical simplicity of alcohol (ethanol), its pharmacology is quite complex. Furthermore, alcohol abuse is often associated with other forms of drug use such as heavy smoking, and barbiturate and benzodiazepine abuse. Co-morbid psychiatric disorders may be present such as depression or phobic anxiety and further complicate the issue. The social aspects of the addiction such as the extent of an alcohol subculture in the social milieu, family disruption, financial status and physical complications affect the treatment both in terms of short-term efficacy and long-term outcome.

The consumption of alcohol is widespread and the safe limits for consumption have recently been revised. The recommended weekly limit is 28 units for men, 21 for women, a unit being roughly a half-pint of beer, a glass of wine or a single measure of spirits. Alcohol problems are age-related, with over a quarter of young males encountering some, usually transient, difficulties. Multiple serious life problems associated with alcohol use (a practical definition of alcoholism) afflict 3–5% of men and up to 1% of women in the UK. But surveys of medical and surgical patients in hospital reveal much higher rates because of the frequency of physical complaints associated with heavy drinking.

Drinking patterns fluctuate markedly over time making it more difficult to assess putative treatments. In any year, the patient will experience bouts of heavy uncontrolled drinking but also episodes of relative abstinence. Only a minority pursue an inexorable downward course (the 'skid-row' alcoholic), most maintaining some precarious foothold in family and employment. Few return to controlled social drinking so that the primary aim of treatment for most should be encouragement of total abstinence. The first step in treatment, however, may be detoxification.

Alcohol Detoxification

Weaning the alcohol abuser off alcohol is only the first and often the easiest step in the management. Detoxification provides symptomatic relief from the withdrawal symptoms, it prevents withdrawal complications and it should facilitate the long-term treatment aimed at encouraging abstinence.

Detoxification is essentially controlled withdrawal using prescribed medication which is cross-tolerant with and can substitute for the alcohol (Table 12.1). The benzodiazepines are the usual drugs used but in the UK and some other countries, chlormethiazole is preferred by some therapists.

Diazepam and chlordiazepoxide have a long duration of action because they are metabolised in the liver to long-acting active metabolites, mainly nordiazepam. However, in patients with liver impairment, oxazepam and lorazepam are preferable because they undergo a simpler metabolic pattern, less affected by liver malfunctioning. A typical regimen is to administer 10 mg of diazepam or 50 mg of chlordiazepoxide orally several times a day as needed, usually for three to four days, by which time the patient has usually lost his abstinence symptoms of tremor, nausea, insomnia and sweating. Some advocate higher initial doses until the patient is mildly sedated and then no further medication unless essential. The latter strategy usually entails lower total drug dosage than the former.

Chlormethiazole is also cross-tolerant to alcohol, although its precise mode of action is unclear. The usual dosage regimen involves giving 500 mg three or

Table 12.1 Drugs used in alcohol withdrawal

Phase	Drug
I Acute detoxification	
Cross-tolerant	Benzodiazepines Chlormethiazole
Symptomatic relief	Propranolol Clonidine
Replacement/prevention	Multivitamins
Contraindicated	Antipsychotics Tricyclic antidepressants
II Maintenance	
Alcohol-sensitising	Disulfiram Calcium Carbimide

four times a day for a few days with a tapering schedule. The drug should not be used beyond five days because of the risk of transferring the dependence to chlormethiazole. Furthermore, the combination of alcohol and chlormethiazole can lead to fatal respiratory depression. Therefore, it should not be used in alcoholic patients who fail to stay abstinent.

The complications of alcohol withdrawal are withdrawal seizures, usually occurring within 72 hours of abstinence and delirium tremens which usually supervenes later than this. A history of withdrawal seizures should alert the therapist to using large doses of diazepam or chlormethiazole or prescribing phenytoin 100 mg thrice daily for about five days.

Other drugs used in withdrawal include propranolol for patients with severe tremor and clonidine for hypertension. Paraldehyde, chloral hydrate and the barbiturates are now obsolescent if not obsolete. Vitamins are usually given routinely to prevent uncommon but serious neurological complications such as Wernicke's encephalopathy. Although thiamine is the vitamin mainly involved, multivitamin therapy is usually given, the first few doses by injection.

Antipsychotic and antidepressant drugs are not appropriate in alcohol withdrawal and may increase the risk of withdrawal fits. They may be indicated after withdrawal to treat psychotic and depressive symptoms respectively. After withdrawal, patients should be encouraged to enter a programme of alcoholism treatment.

Maintenance of Abstinence

In the pursuit of this aim, alcohol-sensitising drugs have been used for many years, but still their utility is a matter of controversy. The only one available in the UK is disulfiram but calcium carbimide is prescribable elsewhere. These drugs produce irreversible inhibition of aldehyde dehydrogenase, one of the enzymes in the breakdown pathway of alcohol. Aldehyde accumulates so that alcohol produces quite promptly a characteristic syndrome with hypotension, racing pulse, flushing, panting, headache, nausea and vomiting. The effects wear off as the new enzyme is synthesised.

Disulfiram itself has a range of unwanted effects including lethargy, fatigue and drowsiness. More rarely, an acute encephalopathy or frank psychosis has been reported. Liver damage may rarely supervene. If a large amount of alcohol is taken the subsequent interaction can be hazardous or even fatal, with severe hypotension and cardiac arrhythmias. Interactions with other drugs are also well-documented, phenytoin, sympathomimetic agents, tricyclic antidepressants, antipsychotic drugs and some forms of chemotherapy (e.g. metronidazole) being implicated.

Because of these potential complications, disulfiram should only be given to heavy drinkers who definitely wish to abstain, agree to take the drug regularly, and have no co-morbid psychiatric disorder. The dosage is 250 mg orally once each night and as it has a slow onset of action, it must be taken at least 12 hours before the patient is exposed to risk. Some therapists insist on a trial administration of alcohol to demonstrate to the patient the nature of the reaction and to obviate undue sensitivity.

Disulfiram therapy can be interpreted in terms of learning theory in that it replaces the delayed with the immediate consequences of drinking alcohol, and therefore should deter drinking. However, the efficacy of the treatment depends on total compliance of the patient in taking the disulfiram regularly. Compliance can be checked by detecting the metabolic products of disulfiram and regular monitoring helps to maintain compliance. It can further be improved by mobilising the assistance of a concerned relative or friend who can supervise the drug administration. The use of disulfiram should therefore be a part of a planned, comprehensive programme of psychological and social rehabilitation. Nevertheless, if a heavy drinker makes the conscious decision to resume drinking, he or she merely stops taking his tablets. Implant formulations have been advocated but are regarded by most experts as too dangerous, if the patient does resume alcohol ingestion. Finally, some patients become acclimatised to mild disulfiram-alcohol reactions and may drink steadily almost with impunity.

The benzodiazepines are used not only in abstinence but also in maintenance treatment. They lessen anxiety and aid sleep but are very likely to be abused. Sometimes, the alcoholic transfers dependence from alcohol to the benzodiazepine which is an improvement in physical safety. But too often, the heavy drinker combines alcohol and benzodiazepine drugs because of the potentiation of effects.

Other drugs which have been studied as abstinence enhancers include bromocriptine, the selective serotonin re-uptake inhibitor, antidepressants, and the opioid antagonist, naltrexone.

Psychological Management of Alcohol-related Problems

The models of treatment for alcohol misuse have often been polarised into disease versus behavioural but in clinical practice, an integrated approach is often used with most success.

Many people consuming excessive amounts of alcohol have no desire to change their habits and so motivation to change is a key concept in this field. It has been suggested that there are at least four stages in this process (Table 12.2): pre-contemplation, contemplation, action and maintenance. Progress is not smooth and a failed attempt may lead back to stage 1. People may remain at the contemplation stage for minutes or years but success has been shown to be more likely if someone is prepared for action (stage 3). Even during maintenance (stage 4), vigilance is required as clients may relapse after several months (or even years) of apparent success.

Treatment Approaches

A recent review examined 34 treatment approaches in controlled clinical trials with either a randomised or a matched comparison group design. They found

Table 12.2   Stages in the motivation to change process

Stage	
1. Pre-contemplation	No intention to change
2. Contemplation	Costs and benefits appraised Ability to cope with change assessed
3. Action	Pledge made Positive steps taken
4. Maintenance	Prevention of relapse

Table 12.3   Effective psychological treatments for alcohol problems

Social skills training
Self-control training
Brief motivational counselling
Behavioural marital therapy
Community reinforcement approach
Stress management training

that six treatments showed good evidence of effectiveness and these were largely behavioural approaches (Table 12.3). These will be briefly described but fuller descriptions of all the approaches are given in Holder et al. (1991). It should be pointed out that some widely used methods, e.g. Alcoholics Anonymous, have not been subjected to rigorous scientific study and so insufficient evidence exists by which to judge their effectiveness.

Social skills training. The client is taught (usually in a group) specific behavioural skills for initiating and maintaining interpersonal relationships. This may involve assertiveness training.

Self-control training. Specific self-management skills are taught to help the client reduce or avoid alcohol consumption. Strategies include specific goal-setting, self-monitoring, rate reduction, self-reinforcement, functional analysis and learning alternative ways of coping.

Brief motivational counselling. This involves one to three sessions of motivational feedback and advice. The client is given an assessment of alcohol-related impairment and is advised to change his/her drinking pattern.

Behavioural marital therapy. The aim is to improve communication and problem-solving skills between the client and spouse and to increase the exchange of positive reinforcement.

Community reinforcement approach. The broad-spectrum behavioural approach seeks to change the client's environment to make abstinence more rewarding than drinking. Daily doses of disulfiram are administered by a significant other (the spouse). Strategies involve job-finding, problem-solving, improving relationships and increasing involvement in non-alcohol related leisure activities.

Stress management training. The client is taught methods to reduce personal tension and stress, e.g. relaxation techniques, systematic desensitisation.

The community reinforcement approach which combines drug and behavioural treatment was shown to be more effective than either oral or implant disulfiram alone but giving the partner responsibility for administering the drug may improve compliance with oral medication. Structured behavioural techniques were also found to be more successful than cognitive therapy and teaching positive skills was better than negative behavioural techniques like chemical or electrical aversion therapy. This is in agreement with a study of therapist style. It was found that a *client-centred* style in which the therapist tried to elicit and reflect the client's own concerns was more effective than a *directive* style in which clients were urged didactically to accept a label of alcoholism and to seek treatment. Other psychological techniques may prove effective but require more investigation before being widely or routinely used, e.g. covert sensitisation, behaviour contracting and other non-behavioural forms of marital and cognitive therapy. Cue exposure is a useful technique which may be incorporated in various forms of treatment, e.g. self-control training.

Treatment for alcohol-related problems has been moving steadily away from in-patient programmes since a lack of evidence for improved efficacy over community or out-patient alcoholic clinics has been repeatedly confirmed. Brief interventions have become more common and seem to be effective in reducing drinking. The first interview has been shown to be of prime importance to establish good rapport and sustain and raise the client's self-confidence in their own ability to follow sensible advice on drinking.

In conclusion, there is an abundance of information now on the successful treatment of heavy drinking. However there is a need for more education and improved detection. Significant progress might be made by integrating the best pharmacological and behavioural approaches in those with severe alcohol-related problems.

DRUG DEPENDENCE

A wide range of drugs are misused both within and outwith the therapeutic context. The main agents are the opioids (e.g. diamorphine (heroin) and methadone), the stimulants (cocaine and amphetamine), the sedatives (barbiturates and benzodiazepines), the hallucinogens (LSD and mescaline) and cannabis. Drugs are used in the treatment of several of these conditions and their use is outlined below. Apart from symptomatic relief, drugs are used either as replacement therapy in a detoxification or maintenance programme or as antagonists in an attempt to block positive reinforcement (Table 12.4).

Table 12.4   The use of drugs in the treatment of drug dependence

Replacement	
Heroin	Methadone
Cigarette smoking	Nicotine

Antagonist	
Heroin	Naltrexone
Cocaine	Desipramine

Opioid Dependence

As with alcohol abuse, management of patients (clients) with opioid dependence focuses on two main areas, detoxification and maintenance of a controlled dose or abstinence.

The withdrawal schedules for opioids usually involve the administration of oral methadone in decreasing dosage. However, some mildly dependent patients can be withdrawn without pharmacological aids. The usual preparation where a substitute is needed is oral methadone mixture 1 mg/ ml. This is long lasting, effective and unlikely to be injected. Dihydrocodeine tablets are an alternative but need frequent administration. The dosage of a substitute needs careful appraisal, the goal being to transfer the patient to the minimal dose necessary to avoid withdrawal symptoms, typically nausea, vomiting, diarrhoea, restlessness, insomnia, bodily pains, sweating, yawning, running eyes and nose with sneezing and dilated pupils and gooseflesh. A careful drug history will provide an estimate of the appropriate dosage of methadone which is then titrated against the early and mild symptoms of withdrawal such as pupillary dilatation, rapid pulse beat, and sweating. The methadone is then withdrawn by small daily reductions from this initial dose. Often reduction can be effected more rapidly at first with smaller decremental steps later. Typically, the initial dosage of 30–40 mg once a day of methadone can be reduced over three to four weeks by 5 mg/week and then from 20 mg/ day in smaller doses. This rather protracted withdrawal can be accelerated somewhat if the client is in hospital. Once free of opioids, intensive treatment and psychosocial programmes are needed to maintain abstinence.

Other medications have been used, mainly symptomatically. These include propranolol which is useful for palpitations and bodily anxiety, and diphenoxylate and atropine (Lomotil) to combat diarrhoea. The latter is sometimes combined with thioridazine which has sedative actions. Benzodiazepines have sometimes been used but they have an addiction potential in their own right. In hospital, a few days' course may lessen severe anxiety but the risk of dependence, often with intravenous use, precludes routine treatment.

Clonidine is an alpha$_2$ adrenergic agonist that antagonises noradrenergic arousal mechanisms in the brain. The withdrawal syndrome is hypothesised to stem from noradrenergic overactivity so clonidine has been used with some success in opioid withdrawal. Later, clonidine, itself, has to be tapered off to avoid rebound rises in blood pressure. Lofexidine is a newly-introduced similar compound. Rapid detoxification by combining an opioid antagonist such as naltrexone with clonidine has been found effective in appropriate circumstances.

Methadone Maintenance

Methadone is a synthetic opioid agonist which acts mainly on the μ receptors which are particularly involved in analgesia and euphoria and which show rapid tolerance and dependence. Methadone is well absorbed after oral administration and can easily substitute for heroin. It is given to addicts in a liquid non-injectable form to help the client to stop taking other opioids, particularly those taken by intravenous injection. By this means, harm minimisation is effected, the client stabilises his opioid use and is in regular contact with treatment services. As methadone has a plasma half-life of 16–24 hours in opioid-naive individuals and 24–48 hours in chronic users, the client can be maintained on a single, usually morning dose. The process of methadone maintenance can be rationalised as a breathing space while the client readjusts his or her attitudes, motivations, and ultimately, life-style. In the USA, it has the added attraction that it can be legally prescribed, unlike heroin. Oral methadone results in much less euphoria than injected heroin, and, of course, all the attendant pathology of injecting is avoided.

The usual daily dose of methadone is 30–40 mg, although a few clients need more than this. At one time, high doses were used with the intention of blocking the effects of heroin administered illicitly, but prolonged dependence results, and this procedure is not now commonly used.

The methadone is issued daily to regulate its use and to discourage illicit dissemination of spare supplies. Doling it out at the clinic is the best procedure but arrangements for a daily issue from a pharmacist can be made. Counselling and other forms of therapy are essential, otherwise the treatment degenerates into mere drug provision, and the client may start to combine his regular methadone with his irregular heroin. Realistic goals should be set and a timetable agreed for a tapering regimen with withdrawal from the methadone. One such timetable involves a year's maintenance on methadone followed by withdrawal over three to six months. A few clinics prescribe injectable diamorphine (heroin) in an attempt to stabilise chaotic opioid injectors. However, this should not be prolonged indefinitely, not least on the grounds of expense.

Other opioid substitutes have been tried. One, levo-alpha-acetylmethadol (LAMM) has a duration of action of 72 hours so it can be given every few days. Buprenorphine, a partial agonist, has also been tried with some success.

Naltrexone Blockade

An alternative strategy is to try and block the effects of injected heroin. Naltrexone is an opioid antagonist with a half-life of about 72 hours. Side-effects are infrequent but include yawning, stretching, and mental stimulation. There is no withdrawal syndrome on cessation. High doses are associated with abnormal liver function tests. Studies evaluating naltrexone (and other blockers, for that matter), have not been very encouraging, mainly because of poor patient compliance. Nevertheless, some special groups, such as highly motivated professionals may show better results.

Stimulant Abuse

Cocaine is a drug of abuse which is currently in widespread, almost epidemic use, in the USA. Its abuse is spreading throughout Europe especially in the 'free base' form which is suitable for smoking, and which is extremely addictive because of its rapid penetration to the brain with an immediate 'high'. 'Crack' is ready-to-use low-priced cocaine in its free base form.

The psychotropic effects of cocaine are mainly mediated through the dopaminergic reward systems in the brain. Cocaine is a powerful re-uptake inhibitor, thus enhancing dopaminergic activity such as reward mechanisms.

The pharmacological treatment of cocaine abuse can be split into four areas:

1. *Acute* administration of drugs intended to lessen craving. These include amantadine, bromocriptine and L-dopa, all of which are dopaminergic compounds, although their mode of action varies. Single-dose placebo-controlled cross-over trials have suggested some efficacy. Open studies of two to three weeks duration have been encouraging: craving is lessened and use of cocaine is decreased.
2. *Symptomatic* relief of withdrawal symptoms can be given to some extent by antipsychotic drugs such as chlorpromazine and fluphenazine, and/or

benzodiazepines. Addicts often self-administer a benzodiazepine in an attempt to ameliorate the 'crash' symptoms of acute withdrawal.

3. *Chronic* administration of antidepressants is advocated in order to lessen the risks of relapse after withdrawal. The rationale is that these drugs block the re-uptake of monoamine neurotransmitters, reducing the brain's sensitivity to cocaine. Several trials have shown that agents such as desipramine significantly reduce cocaine use and craving but the clinical effect is small in practice. The onset of action is usually delayed 10–20 days during which time up to a third of patients may drop out of treatment.

4. *Co-morbid* psychiatric disorders such as depression, both unipolar and manic-depressive, may need treatment in their own right, usually with antidepressants or lithium.

The amphetamines are actually more widely abused than cocaine but receive less publicity. Their pharmacology is similar and the drug treatments listed above are usually appropriate as well.

OTHER DRUGS OF ABUSE

Phencyclidine, cannabis and the hallucinogens are associated with toxic effects and possible withdrawal phenomena. Symptomatic treatment may be needed as appropriate but specific medication is not available.

Nicotine Dependence

Cigarette smoking has caused more suffering to Western populations than all other forms of addiction combined. The threat of death, however, is outweighed in a quarter of adults by the pleasure provided by smoking and by the undoubted dependence-inducing properties of nicotine.

Giving up smoking has always proved difficult with a high relapse rate. Furthermore, patterns of smoking vary substantially and may reflect different underlying mechanisms. Consequently, techniques suitable for helping some smokers desist may be ineffective in others. Sex differences seem important in smoking mechanisms and withdrawal.

Among the older remedies, usually available without prescription, are to be found:

1. Silver acetate lozenges — sucking them makes cigarette smoke taste bitter so an aversion should be produced. No evidence of efficacy exists.
2. Lobeline sulphate which is a nicotine antagonist of sorts, and should block the pleasurable effects of smoking. Efficacy is unestablished.

3. Scopolamine is an anticholinergic agent (antimuscarinic), which seems also to lessen nicotine's effect. It is available as transdermal patches, but treatment of nicotine withdrawal is usually started with an injection together with chlorpromazine. Some preliminary evidence for efficacy exists.

4. Clonidine, the alpha$_2$ adrenergic compound can also help alleviate withdrawal symptoms including craving, anxiety, restlessness and irritability. Longer-term efficacy has not been demonstrated consistently.

Nicotine replacement therapy is based on the premise that cigarette smoking has two broad components, the behavioural repertoire which is secondary conditioned behaviour, and the pharmacological nicotine dependence. By separating these components and extinguishing the behaviour first, better abstinence rates should be attained. Thus, the nicotine from the cigarette smoke is replaced by some other form of nicotine delivery, to provide a form of maintenance therapy.

Nicotine-containing chewing gum has been the most thoroughly evaluated. Careful supervised use of the gum in a special clinic approximately doubles long-term abstinence rates from 15–20% to 30–40%. In primary care settings or in self-administered unsupervised use, success rates are less impressive. The client should be aware of the rationale for nicotine replacement, know of its effects, use a reasonable amount for a sufficient period of time and start using the gum only after stopping smoking completely.

Other forms of nicotine replacement are now available or being actively developed. Transdermal skin patches provide a steady background nicotine level; nasal spray and nicotine vapour provide bursts of nicotine more closely mimicking the effects of a cigarette. Various combinations are also being evaluated.

More recently the 5-HT$_{1A}$ partial agonist, buspirone, has been shown to be as effective as transdermal nicotine with fewer adverse effects. The drug is allowed to reach a steady state before smoking is stopped.

PSYCHOLOGICAL MANAGEMENT OF DRUG DEPENDENCE

Medications only treat some aspects of drug dependence and they cannot achieve the critical therapeutic goal of changing behaviour. However, by blocking the reinforcing effects of drugs, reducing their withdrawal symptoms and thus lengthening periods of remission, they can provide conditions under which psychotherapeutic treatments can be implemented more successfully.

Motivation to change is as important as with alcohol problems, but because of the illegality of many abused drugs, treatment may be imposed by the authorities. The first level of psychological management is advice and this may be all that is necessary to encourage some people to abstain. However, the majority will need more structured help. Psychotherapeutic techniques are numerous and similar to those employed in alcohol problems but the area has far fewer controlled studies delineating effectiveness and so far no particular approach has been shown to be superior. It has been suggested that brief, less intensive approaches may be sufficient for clients without significant accompanying psychopathology, but for those with concurrent psychiatric disorders more elaborate forms of psychotherapeutic intervention may be necessary. It has been shown that heavier users of cocaine may differentially respond to more structured and directive approaches and that the outcome of methadone maintenance is strongly mediated by the psychosocial aspects of treatment. It seems likely that for the majority of drug users, an integrated scheme similar to the community reinforcement approach, incorporating counselling for interpersonal conflict, behavioural techniques to encourage extinction of drug seeking and to prevent relapse, as well as altering the social environment of the individual, would prove most effective. Pharmacological interventions should be incorporated into the programme as appropriate.

Even in more straightforward, legal forms of addiction, e.g. smoking, medication alone cannot induce abstention and can only result in a reduction of consumption in motivated individuals. The effective use of medications whether as replacement, e.g. nicotine or as antagonist, e.g. naltrexone, depends on other concurrent mechanisms to change behaviour. Consequently, the most positive outcomes appear to have been reached with a combination of psychotherapeutic and pharmacological treatments.

SUMMARY

Alcohol is the most commonly abused drug and there is a need for more education and improved detection of alcohol-related problems. A wide range of drugs are misused for their various properties. Motivation to change is very important and intervention is unlikely to succeed without commitment by the client. The first interview is very important in establishing good rapport and reinforcing the client's ability to tackle these problems. Drug and psychological treatment are best combined in an out-patient clinic setting. Medication can help to control withdrawal symptoms in detoxification and to maintain abstinence. Structured behavioural treatments are most effective and a broad-spectrum approach with the aim of enabling the client to change their social environment is likely to be most successful.

FURTHER READING

Ball, J.C. and Ross, A. (1991) *The Effectiveness of Methadone Maintenance Treatment*. Springer-Verlag, New York.

Benowitz, N.L. (1993) Nicotine replacement therapy. What has been accomplished — Can we do better? *Drugs* **45**, 157–170.

Carroll, K.M., Rounsaville, B.J., Gordon, L.T. et al. (1994) Psychotherapy and pharmacotherapy for ambulatory cocaine abusers. *Archives of General Psychiatry* **51**, 177–187.

Castaneda, R. and Cushman, P. (1989) Alcohol withdrawal: a review of clinical management. *Journal of Clinical Psychiatry* **50**, 278–284.

Commentaries (1994) Comments on the WHO report 'Brief interventions for alcohol problems': a summary and some international comments. *Addiction* **89**, 657–678.

Gossop, M., Griffiths, P., Powis, B. and Strang, J. (1994) Cocaine: patterns of use, route of administration, and severity of dependence. *British Journal of Psychiatry* **164**, 660–664.

Henningfield, J.E. and Singleton, E.G. (1994) Managing drug dependence. Psychotherapy or pharmacotherapy? *CNS Drugs* **1**, 317–322.

Hodgson, R.J. (1989) Resisting temptation: psychological analysis. *British Journal of Addiction* **84**, 251–257.

Holder, H., Longabaugh, R., Miller, W.R. and Rubonis, A.V. (1991). The cost effectiveness of treatment for alcoholism: first approximation. *Journal of Studies on Alcohol* **52**, 517–540.

Levin, F.R. and Lehman, A.F. (1991) Metanalysis of desipramine as an adjunct in the treatment of cocaine addiction. *Journal of Clinical Psychopharmacology* **11**, 374–378.

Marlett, G.A. and Gordon, J.R. (1985) *Relapse Prevention: Maintenance Strategies in the Treatment of Addictive Behaviours*. Guilford Press, New York.

McLellan, A.T., Arndt, I.O., Metzger, D.S., Woody, G.E. and O'Brien, C.P. (1993). The effects of psychosocial services in substance abuse treatment. *Journal of the American Medical Association* **269**, 1953–1959.

Miller, W.R. and Sovereign, R.G. (1988) The check-up: a model for early intervention in addictive behaviors. In *Addictive Behaviors: Prevention and Early Intervention* (Loberg, T., Miller, W.R., Nathan, P.E. and Marlatt, G.A., eds). Swetz and Zeitlinger, Amsterdam.

Morgenstern, J. and McCrady, B.S. (1992) Curative factors in alcohol and drug treatment: behavioural and disease model perspectives. *British Journal of Addiction* **87**, 901–912.

Prochaska, J.O. and DiClemente, C.C. (1986) Toward a comprehensive model of change. In *Treating Addictive Behaviors: Processes of Change* (Miller, W.R. and Heather, N. (eds). Plenum Press, New York.

Satel, S.L., Kosten, T.R. Schuckit, M.A. and Fischman, M.W. (1993) Should protracted withdrawal from drugs be included in DSM-IV? *American Journal of Psychiatry* **150**, 695–704.

Steele, T.D., McCann, U.D. and Ricaurte, G.A. (1994) 3,4-methylenedioxymethamphetamine (MDMA, 'ecstasy'): pharmacology and toxicology in animals and humans. *Addiction* **89**, 539–551.

Thom, B., Brown, C., Drummond, C., Edwards, G., Mullan, M. and Taylor, C. (1992) Engaging patients with alcohol problems in treatment: the first consultation. *British Journal of Addiction* **87**, 601–611.

Tang, J.L., Law, M. and Wald, N. (1994) How effective is nicotine replacement therapy in helping people to stop smoking? *British Medical Journal* **308**, 21–23.

Woody, G.E., McLellan, T., Luborsky, L. and O'Brien, C.P. (1987) Twelve-month follow-up of psychotherapy for opiate dependence. *American Journal of Psychiatry* **144**, 590–596.

Chapter 13

DRUG TREATMENT OF OTHER DISORDERS

In this chapter, we review several groups of drugs which are used in the management of a variety of common and important conditions. The use of drugs may be as an adjunct, as in eating disorders, or it may be the mainstay of treatment, as in the case of the anticonvulsants. Particular emphasis, as in previous chapters, is placed on the interactions between drug and non-drug modalities of treatment.

EATING DISORDERS

Obesity

The commonest eating disorder is obesity, a condition with serious adverse effects on health because of its association with diabetes, hypertension and high blood cholesterol. There is clear evidence that reducing weight decreases the risk of these conditions as well as having bonuses in the way of enhanced self-image and personal satisfaction. Nevertheless, as is well-known, reducing weight can be a difficult procedure and a frustrating target to achieve.

The usual definition of being significantly overweight is that the body mass index (BMI = weight in kg/[height in m]^2) is equal to or greater than 30. Such people need to lose about 30 kg, which is equivalent to over 200 000 calories (kcal). As an average calorific requirement is about 2000 calories and low-calorie diets aim at about 1000 calories per day, such a weight loss is going to take over six months. It is important that hopeful weight losers are aware of this simple arithmetic and its implications in terms of required motivations and perseverance.

Bulimia Nervosa

In bulimia nervosa (BN), eating habits are markedly disturbed. The syndrome is characterised by repeated bouts of gross overeating accompanied by various behaviours to control body shape and weight such as extreme dieting, self-induced vomiting and the misuse of laxatives. BN has become a focus of research and therapeutic interest in the past decade. It is a common condition and minor forms often go undetected. Many bulimics are also depressed, although the relationship between depression and the eating disorder is often complex.

Anorexia Nervosa

Anorexia nervosa is characterised by deliberate weight loss induced and/or maintained by the patient (at least 15% below the expected weight). There is an intense fear of gaining weight. It is most common among adolescent girls and young women.

Drug Treatment of Eating Disorders

Obesity

Dietary patterns are deeply ingrained and change is not easily effected Because of this, appetite-reducing drugs have been developed and quite widely used to help patients by reducing their hunger and helping them adhere to a reduced calorific intake. The first such drug was amphetamine which was introduced into medical practice over 50 years ago. Originally, the racemic mixture (DL) was used but this was later largely supplanted by the dextro isomer, dexamphetamine. During the 1950s and into the 1960s, dexamphetamine was widely used as an appetite-suppressant and also to elevate the low-grade depressions often complained of by obese individuals both on and off a diet. Unfortunately, the amphetamines have pronounced stimulant and euphoriant properties, resulting in two forms of inappropriate use: firstly, many obese individuals took regular but still therapeutic doses of amphetamine as a 'pick-me-up', but failed to lose weight; secondly, high doses were used by obese and non-obese people and amphetamine became a very commonly abused drug. Problems with amphetamine have continued throughout. Amphetamines are available illicitly for both oral, and more ominously, intravenous use.

Since then, a range of appetite-suppressant drugs have been developed, some rather akin to the amphetamines but others acting differently, with distinct pharmacological and clinical properties. Those currently available fall into two broad groupings, those acting on catecholamine systems, and those working through 5-HT mechanisms. As the control of appetite is complex, yet further groups of drug treatments are feasible. *Amphetamine* acts by increasing dopaminergic and noradrenergic neurotransmission, which in turn reduces appetite through hypothalamic mechanisms. *Diethylpropion* has less stimulant activity than amphetamine and has proven efficacy in reducing weight, at least in the short-term. As with most appetite-suppressants, individual variation in efficacy is quite marked. Adverse effects include insomnia, are less than with amphetamine, as is the risk of dependence and abuse. *Phentermine* is very similar and is usually administered as a sustained-release preparation. *Mazindol* is a potent appetite-suppressant but can produce nervousness and insomnia. Dry mouth, sweating and constipation have also been reported. It has only low dependence and abuse potential. There is some evidence that *phenylpropanolamine*, a common constituent of cough and cold remedies has useful anorectic properties but it is mildly stimulant and may be abused on occasion.

Drugs acting on central 5-HT pathways can also reduce appetite. *Fenfluramine* is a racemic mixture of the D- and L-forms and it acts by stimulating the release of 5-HT and blocking its re-uptake. It also affects dopamine release. It is not stimulant, indeed, if anything, it is somewhat depressant. It has an active metabolite, norfenfluramine. Fenfluramine has a potent anorectic effect in both normal volunteers and obese patients. A large number of placebo-controlled trials have shown a definite effect in reducing weight. Controlled studies have also shown that it is more effective than psychotherapy or behaviour modification but that fenfluramine can be profitably given in conjunction with behavioural treatments. Drowsiness and fatigue may be reported early in treatment but stimulant properties are absent. Nevertheless, abrupt withdrawal of fenfluramine treatment can precipitate a severe depression, so it should always be tapered off. *Dexfenfluramine* is the D-isomer alone and is more selective in its actions on 5-HT mechanisms. It seems to have a particular effect on reducing carbohydrate intake, especially taken in the form of snacks, but this remains open to debate. Several quite long-term trials (one year) have established its efficacy in obesity. When patients are randomly allocated to receive either 15 mg of dexfenfluramine or placebo as well as a calorie-restricted diet, weight loss is significantly greater in those on active drug, with more than twice as many patients losing 10% or more of their body weight than placebo-recipients. However, the time-course is similar: most weight loss occurs in the first six months, then weight plateaus until drug withdrawal when it increases again particularly in those treated with the active drug. Adverse events are unremarkable.

Fluoxetine is an antidepressant of the selective serotonin re-uptake type (see p. 138). It causes weight loss in depressed patients but mainly those who are overweight. Clinical trials have shown it to have efficacy as an appetite-suppressant but its use is mainly in bulimic patients. The adverse events are mainly insomnia, drowsiness (apparently paradoxical but individual responses vary), nausea and diarrhoea.

Official viewpoints are unsympathetic to the use of appetite-suppressants. For example, the British National Formulary regards them 'as of no real value in the treatment of obesity as they do not improve the long-term outlook'. The alternative opinion is that they are useful adjuncts to dietary advice and behavioural treatments. Many adverse opinions are a relic of the excessive reliance on amphetamine-like compounds 30 years ago, together with a therapeutic Calvinistic view that obese people have only themselves to blame. Conversely, efficacy is usually limited, and long-term usage is not justified.

Bulimia Nervosa

Fluoxetine has been extensively evaluated in the management of bulimic disorders and is now licensed in some countries for this indication. It is often quite effective but should be combined with appropriate behavioural management.

Anorexia Nervosa

A range of drugs has been used to treat AN. Antipsychotic drugs such as chlorpromazine have been advocated but controlled data are sparse. A serotonin antagonist, cyproheptadine, has been tried but without great success. Antidepressants are needed if any mood disorder is present, depression being a common problem. However, lithium should be avoided in anorectic patients because they are often vomiting, or inducing diarrhoea with aperients, or have electrolyte imbalances.

Psychological Treatment of Eating Disorders

Obesity

Excess weight seems to result from a combination of factors. Obese individuals both under-report their caloric intake and overestimate their energy expenditure from physical activity and so careful attention must be paid to the assessment and then modification of eating behaviour. However, it has been suggested that some people are born with a low resting metabolic rate and that there is a genetic predisposition to obesity despite normal caloric intake. This knowledge has led to a reduction of emphasis on ideal weight attainment and the adoption of the reasonable weight criterion. This criterion is dependent on the presence of current health problems and/or a significant family history of obesity-related illness but a reduction in initial weight of as little as 10% may result in significant improvements in both physical and psychological health.

Table 13.1   Behavioural methods of weight control

1. Record eating behaviour	—	amount
		type
		frequency
2. Stimulus control		
3. Slow rate of eating		
4. Increase activity levels		
5. Record weight loss	—	goal setting
6. Elicit social support		

Weight reduction may be achieved by very-low-calorie diets or by modifying eating habits. Behavioural methods of weight control are summarised in Table 13.1. These methods are successful in achieving weight loss during the treatment period but most clients regain during the maintenance period. A programme of regular exercise helps to combat this and is an important adjunct in long-term weight control.

Binge eating is common among the obese and chronic dieters and it has been suggested that this group could form a separate diagnostic category, known as 'binge eating disorder'. These individuals differ from those with BN because they do not compensate for their overeating by other measures of weight control, i.e. vomiting, laxative abuse. However, it is likely that they would benefit from treatment methods used in BN.

Bulimia Nervosa

In contrast to AN, there are numerous treatment studies of BN. Various psychological approaches have been studied (Table 13.2) and all have shown some efficacy. It has been suggested that a stepped care or sequential approach should be adopted. For subclinical disorder or for new cases of short duration, simple educational procedures focusing on nutritional management and self-monitoring may be sufficient. Those who do not respond may require the introduction of more behavioural techniques and more severe cases will require a more complex therapeutic approach. Group treatment often incorporates a variety of techniques and may have very different orientations. However meta-analyses have shown no definite advantage of one therapeutic approach over another.

One meta-analysis showed psychological treatments to be superior to drug treatments, but this only included 15 publications up to December 1985 and so was conducted before the advent of many of the new drugs. A more recent meta-analysis found an effect size for group treatment of $+0.75$ but larger

Table 13.2   Psychological approaches used in the treatment of bulimia nervosa

1. Psychoeducation
2. Group psychotherapy
3. Behaviour therapy
4. Supportive-expressive therapy
5. Interpersonal psychotherapy
6. Cognitive behaviour therapy

effect sizes were associated with more intensive therapy and with the addition of other treatment components such as individual therapy. It has been postulated that the group approach may be particularly beneficial to bulimia as shame and secrecy is reduced by shared disclosure but another meta-analysis found no difference between the two approaches. Effect size (+ 1.04) was improved by number of sessions: for the 10 treatments with at least 15 sessions, it became + 1.37.

Cognitive therapy has been claimed to have increased efficacy because it aims to change abnormal attitudes and assumptions about shape and weight in addition to the illness behaviour but this may only be necessary with more severe cases. In studies comparing psychological treatments: cognitive, behaviour, supportive-expressive and interpersonal therapies, all treatments substantially reduce the principal complaint, i.e. frequency of overeating, and improve secondary psychiatric symptoms and social adjustment. Both cognitive behaviour therapy and behaviour therapy are also effective in reducing the frequency of self-induced vomiting but cognitive behaviour therapy is the only treatment to modify attempts to diet and disturbed attitudes to eating, shape and weight. There is also some evidence that improvement with cognitive therapy is maintained at follow-up. It seems likely, therefore, that cognitive behaviour therapy would be the most appropriate treatment for bulimics with a severely disturbed body image. It remains to be determined if it leads to a better long-term outcome.

Anorexia Nervosa

The behavioural treatment of AN consists of refeeding and prevention of purging (vomiting, laxative abuse) in order to restore normal body weight and then the establishment of a healthy eating pattern. However, relapse is common unless some treatment can be targeted at the psychological aspects of the disorder. This has usually focused on individual or family therapy but there are few trials of efficacy. Most studies which have attempted to evaluate psychotherapeutic interventions have also included initial sessions dealing with eating behaviour or dietary advice. Whereas different treatments result in different patterns of improvement, follow-up assessments frequently show overall improvement for any planned intervention compared with a single assessment interview. The conclusion seems to be that a combination treatment in which attention is given both to eating behaviour and psychological health is most effective. It has been suggested that family therapy is particularly effective for younger patients with a shorter duration of illness whereas individual therapy may be more effective in patients with a later onset of illness. Although in-patients have been shown to gain more weight more quickly, this increase is not maintained at one year follow-ups. It seems then that out-patient options are much more cost effective. There is a need for far more controlled trials of psychological intervention strategies in this disorder which results not only in substantial levels of morbidity but also the risk of mortality.

Combination of Drug and Psychological Treatment

In clinical practice, drugs are often a part of the treatment schedule especially in severe cases or in-patients. However, few studies have evaluated the combination objectively.

In obesity, a major study in the USA examined the value of fenfluramine plus phentermine as an adjunct to group behaviour therapy, dietary counselling and exercise over 34 weeks and found the combination to aid weight loss more than non-drug treatment alone. They then continued the drugs in an open-label fashion and found continued efficacy up to 156 weeks. However, when the drugs were stopped, participants regained some of the weight lost. The authors make the point that long-term anorectic medication at variable doses can help clients maintain weight loss.

Two recent studies have evaluated the combination of an antidepressant with some form of psychological treatment in BN. In one, intensive group psychotherapy was found to be superior to imipramine and the combined treatment offered no benefits over psychological treatment in terms of eating behaviour, although it did improve accompanying psychiatric symptoms. The other study examined the effects of desipramine, cognitive behaviour therapy and the combination. Both cognitive behaviour therapy and the combination were superior to the drug given alone for 16 weeks on binge eating and purging behaviour but at 32 weeks only the combined treatment was superior. When medication was stopped, continuing cognitive behaviour therapy appeared to prevent relapse. The conclusion seems to be that the combination of more intensive psychological treatments with longer-term drug therapy is the most effective option but more outcome studies and longer follow-ups are needed to confirm this.

EPILEPSY

Epilepsy is a common and complex group of conditions, and its management is complicated. It is usually the province of neurologists but psychiatrists and psychologists become involved when there are behavioural complications or co-morbid disorders such as depression and paranoid psychosis. The following, therefore, is an outline of drug therapy.

Because it is a chronic condition, the management of epilepsy often becomes complex and polypharmacy may prevail too frequently. Nevertheless, early treatment must be vigorous in order to prevent further fits as much as possible because each fit is capable of causing further cerebral damage. Some patients, however, have only a single attack, some a steady succession of fairly regular attacks, and some a variable pattern with long fit-free periods punctuated by a cluster of attacks. The factors predisposing to a more serious disorder include the presence of a neurological lesion, abnormalities in the EEG, psychosocial difficulties and co-morbid alcohol and substance abuse problems. Perhaps a third of epileptic patients have psychological difficulties but causation may be difficult to disentangle as brain damage, seizure activity and anticonvulsant drug treatment can all be involved.

Anticonvulsant Drugs

Many classes of anticonvulsant drug are used such as the hydantoins, barbiturates, succinimides, benzodiazepines, carbamazepine and sodium valproate. Phenobarbitone, phenytoin and primidone are indicated in the treatment of grand mal (tonic-clonic) epilepsy, carbamazepine in partial seizures (including temporal lobe epilepsy), ethosuximide in petit mal, and the benzodiazepines and sodium valproate in all forms. Many of these drugs are very old so that systematic data relating to efficacy, side effects, dosage, etc. are sparse. Treatment decisions were often determined by experience gained in treatment of the more severe and refractory patients. However, the development of newer anticonvulsants such as lamotrigine has led to a re-examination of treatment principles and in particular the realisation that epilepsy often pursues a relatively benign course.

The mode of action of many anticonvulsants is unclear. They are certainly seizure-suppressants but they may also influence the course of the condition. However, they have a wide range of adverse effects including cognitive impairment so the risk/benefit ratio must be carefully assessed in each patient and set off against the severity of the condition. Single, spontaneous seizures or those occurring during alcohol or drug withdrawal are not generally regarded as indications for long-term anticonvulsant therapy. Even following head-injury or craniotomy where the risk of seizures is fairly high, it may be deemed better to wait than to place everyone on prophylactic medication. The choice of drug is generally governed by the typology of epilepsy outlined earlier, but comparative data within each class are generally lacking. Often the choice of medication resides with individual patient tolerability. Plasma drug concentration estimations are often useful in limiting toxicity.

The patient should be seen regularly to monitor the progress of treatment and the adverse effects load, to improve compliance and to allow counselling on medical and social matters. Some drugs are better tolerated than others: for example, carbamazepine is often preferred because it has fewer unwanted effects than phenytoin or phenobarbitone and also because it often elevates mood somewhat. Newer compounds are not always less toxic; sodium valproate, for example, has significant side-effects. Inevitably, drug regimens tend to become more complex and dosages to creep upwards. After a period without seizures (usually at least two years), anticonvulsant dosage can be very slowly tapered off. During this time, seizures may return, possibly activated by the drug withdrawal. Anxiety and insomnia may occur during withdrawal from phenobarbitone and clonazepam, but not from the other anticonvulsants. Lamotrigine is a new compound whose limits of efficacy are still being explored.

Polypharmacy and high doses can result in unacceptable levels of both somatic and behavioural toxicity. Minor adverse effects include drowsiness, slurring of speech, ataxia, and nausea. Phenytoin may induce gum hyper-trophy and hirsutism. More serious effects include peripheral neuropathy, cerebellar degeneration and osteomalacia. The anticonvulsants interact with many other drugs both by displacement from plasma albumin binding and by induction (increase in activity) of liver metabolising enzymes.

For all these reasons, the management of psychological complications can be complex. Polypharmacy should be rationalised but this must be done slowly to avoid withdrawal fits. Counselling concerning psychosocial problems should be aimed at establishing a sensible, regular life-style. Simple psychological support can sometimes prove unexpectedly beneficial over a range of functions. Seizure frequency may decline and allow a simple anticonvulsant regimen with lower dosages; this may result in a change in personality with a mature, more rational person taking the place of an irritable, hypochondriacal, dependent person.

Psychological Effects of Anticonvulsants

Epilepsy itself can result in neuropsychological impairment. This is very much dependent on the nature of the illness (duration, severity, seizure type) and the age at onset. Thus impairment may be widespread or only transient. Drug treatment may also affect cognition but this must be balanced against reduced seizure frequency which may improve performance. Several older studies suggested differential cognitive effects of various compounds, generally favouring newer drugs like carbamazepine or valproate over the older phenobarbitone and phenytoin. However, recent reviews have emphasised the methodological problems in these studies and the conclusion reached is that although phenobarbitone appears to have relatively more adverse cognitive effects, there is little difference between the other three. Clinically significant cognitive impairment generally occurs only with high doses and polypharmacy and is not generally a problem with a single drug administered within the standard therapeutic range. Individual patients may respond to one particular drug and the influence of psychological factors should not be underestimated. Helping the patient to understand their illness and the influence that both physical and other psychological factors have on their seizures leads to an improvement in quality of life. There is some evidence that relaxation training may help reduce seizure frequency but there are no large-scale, systematically controlled trials of psychological treatments.

Other Uses for Anticonvulsants

Anticonvulsants have a 'stabilising' effect on a range of cerebral functions including emotional and intellectual reactions. Thus, these drugs have been used in a wide range of other indications. Carbamazepine and sodium valproate have been tried with some success in manic-depressive psychosis. Anticonvulsants are sometimes effective in patients characterised by irritability and depression, especially where behavioural problems are sudden and unpredictable. Phenytoin, carbamazepine and primidone often have a dramatic effect in these 'intermittent explosive disorders'. These drugs have also been used to alleviate disturbed behaviour in people with learning disabilities.

PSYCHOTROPIC DRUGS IN THE CONTROL OF AGGRESSION

No drug is specifically licensed for this indication and few have been examined in well-controlled, double-blind trials and even where they have, questions such as optimal length of treatment or comparisons with other potential drug regimes have seldom been addressed. The drugs which are currently used have been developed to treat psychiatric, neurological or medical conditions and not aggressive behaviour *per se* and therefore any beneficial effects on symptoms of aggression are secondary. The antipsychotics are still the standard treatment for controlling aggressive behaviour across diagnoses but they have the disadvantage of serious side-effects such as tardive dyskinesia which make it important to consider alternatives. There is a growing body of evidence that two mood-stabilising drugs used in the treatment of manic-depressive psychosis, lithium and carbamazepine, may have independent effects in controlling aggression and impulsiveness. They seem to be particularly helpful in patients who are unable but wish to control their own aggressive impulses but individuals who indulge their aggressiveness tend to deny the benefits even though they may respond. There is some evidence that beta-blockers may be useful in treating symptoms of aggression and rage associated with brain damage and can be added to antipsychotics to improve such symptoms in schizophrenia. Stimulants have only a limited role in the treatment of aggression associated with minimal brain dysfunction. The evidence for benzodiazepines is much more controversial and they are contraindicated in personality disorder. Although they may be of benefit to some patients, there are no reliable predictive indices and so their use in the control of aggression should be limited to the acute phase during which sedation may be necessary while other longer term treatment is instituted.

Recently, many different strands of work have revealed a link between low levels of central serotonin and impulsive aggressive behaviour and this has led to the experimentation with drugs acting more directly on the serotonin system. Tryptophan, a precursor for serotonin has been shown to have some anti-aggressive effects when added to maintenance anti-psychotic treatment in schizophrenics exhibiting violence or aggression. There is some evidence accruing for a beneficial effect with buspirone, a 5-HT_{1A} partial agonist. This is based largely on case reports but nevertheless it consistently shows a decrease in aggression and self-injury which has been confirmed in one double-blind study. A decrease in anxiety and agitation was reported with no effect on cognitive performance. This latter may be an advantage which can be exploited as it may mean that buspirone can be used in conjunction with psychological therapies such as behaviour modification without impairing learning. A class of drugs which act specifically on the 5-HT_1 receptor, aptly named the serenics — eltoprazine and fluprazine — were developed specifically for their putative anti-aggressive effects. However, results from the first clinical trials have been disappointing and the drugs have not been marketed. Serotonergic antidepressants such as clomipramine and the SSRIs have shown promising preliminary results in the treatment of aggression associated with learning disabilities and personality disorder.

It is important to note that these newer compounds have a delayed onset and exert a gentler, more specific anti-aggressive action not related to sedation which takes some weeks to show an effect. Other more sedative compounds may then be necessary in the interim. The azapirones and SSRIs are relatively safe alternatives with few side-effects and if their efficacy can be demonstrated, they may fast become the treatment of choice in the control of irritable, impulsive aggression.

PSYCHOTROPIC DRUGS AND REPRODUCTION

Premenstrual Tension

A number of bodily and psychological symptoms are reported by many women at certain times in the menstrual cycle. The commonest time is in the luteal phase, that is 7–10 days before the start of menstruation. However, many patterns are seen from woman to woman and even at different phases in the same woman. Typical bodily symptoms include headache, abdominal distension, breast pain and increase in weight. Psychological symptoms comprise anxiety, tension, depression, irritability and inability to concentrate. The usually accepted prevalence in women of child-bearing age is 30–50%. However, the condition is not clearly defined and the prevalence is higher with specific retrospective questioning than with less focused enquiries.

Studies of aetiology, pathogenesis and treatment response are hampered by problems of definition and quantification. Most treatment studies have been unsatisfactory, usually because of lack of adequate placebo control, or failure to standardise concomitant non-drug therapeutic manoeuvres or insufficient duration of study. Psychotropic drugs which have been tried include sedatives, various groups of antidepressants and lithium. Some symptomatic change may be seen, particularly if the woman suffers more chronic rather than episodic affective changes. Some hormonal treatments have their advocates, for example, the synthetic progestogen such as dydrogesterone. Pyridoxine in a dosage of 40 mg twice daily from day 14 of the cycle until menstruation has some effect, particularly where depression is marked. Bromocriptine alters prolactin and may help where breast symptoms are severe. Diuretics may help women who retain fluid towards the end of their menstrual cycle but not all diuretics are of equal efficacy: spironolactone is generally preferred.

Hormonal Replacement Therapy

In both sexes, physical and mental symptoms occurring in middle life have been attributed to endocrine changes. This is particularly so for women after the menopause. Rigorous studies of symptom patterns and treatment response suggest that a few symptoms can be confidently ascribed to menopausal changes. Hot flushes and night sweats are more common at the time of the menopause or shortly afterwards. Minor psychological symptoms such as impaired concentration, anxiety and lack of confidence occur about the same time but aching breasts and low back pain decline steadily in the years following the menopause. Oestrogen replacement lessens flushes and sweating, and reduces osteoporosis and loss of collagen in the skin. It has some protective effect against cardiovascular disease but may slightly increase the risk of cancer of the breast and womb. Hormone replacement therapy, therefore, is not without its critics but many women find it helpful and experience a sense of normality and even well-being, instead of vague dysphorias. In addition, psychological support can be provided at the menopause clinic by the doctor or nurse.

Pregnancy and Puerperium

Drug treatments need special consideration in these contexts for several different reasons, including the effects of drugs on the pregnant mother and foetus, the administration of psychotropic drugs during labour, and the use of such drugs during breast-feeding.

In pregnancy, the general rule is to minimise the use of drugs believed safe and to avoid the use of drugs believed unsafe. However, these categories are often not absolute. In addition, the predictability of animal tests is far from perfect and epidemiological data in humans may be sparse. The first three months of pregnancy is the time of greatest risk. If a woman on psychotropic medication becomes pregnant, the need for the drug should be carefully reviewed and it should be discontinued unless there is a clear need for continuing the medication. Later in pregnancy, if medication has been continued, the dose should be lowered if possible to lessen the likelihood of withdrawal in the baby.

Lithium is the drug which has caused greatest concern. Up to 10% of the offspring of mothers maintained on this drug show congenital malformations, usually cardiovascular in type. Heart valve abnormalities are especially common. If a woman taking lithium wishes to become pregnant, the drug should be withdrawn over two to three months and the patient monitored for possible signs of relapse. Any woman who conceives while taking lithium should have the drug stopped immediately. If this is impossible because of the patient's mental condition, the dose of lithium should be kept low and the baby carefully monitored, e.g. using ultrasound. When labour starts, the lithium should be stopped and resumed later.

Benzodiazepines accumulate in the fetus and can result in the 'floppy infant syndrome' on birth, with the baby being hypotonic, with depressed respiration and poor suckling.

All of the major classes of psychotropic drugs can pass into the breast milk of women taking these drugs at therapeutic levels. However, the milk/plasma ratios that are quoted are often single estimations only, and more systematic data are needed. The pharmacokinetics of drugs in the neonate and infant are often unclear but as a general principle, babies metabolise drugs less slowly than adults so that even small amounts in the breast milk may have marked effects in the baby. In addition, the effects of psychotropic drugs on the developing brain are largely unknown. For all these reasons, most investigators urge caution and recommend that women needing psychotropic medication should not breast-feed.

SUMMARY

Eating disorders are being increasingly recognised in the general population. The use of drugs to control obesity has caused problems in the past and the emphasis now is on behavioural methods of weight control. Behavioural treatment is also important to restore normal weight and eating patterns in AN but other interventions such as family therapy may be necessary to maintain improvement. Both SSRIs and CBT have proved effective in BN.

The management of epilepsy centres on anticonvulsant drugs but psychological factors should not be underestimated. Support and a regular life-style are very important.

Drugs are often used in the control of aggression. Antipsychotics, mood stabilisers and beta-blockers have all shown some effectiveness. Newer drugs acting on serotonin such as buspirone and the SSRIs are currently being evaluated.

Premenstrual tension and menopausal symptoms can usually be treated by manipulating hormones although if psychological symptoms predominate, antidepressants may be indicated. Drug treatment should be minimised during pregnancy and breast-feeding.

FURTHER READING

Aggression

Baumeister, A., Todd, M.E. and Sevin, J.A. (1993) Efficacy and specificity of pharmacological therapies for behavioral disorders in persons with mental retardation. *Clinical Neuropharmacology* **16**, 271–294.

Bond, A.J. (1993) Prospects of anti-aggressive drugs. In *The Science and Psychiatry of Violence* (Thompson, C. and Cowen, P., eds). Butterworth-Heinemann, Oxford, pp. 147–170.

Coccaro, E.F., Kramer, E., Zemishlany, Z. et al. (1990) Pharmacologic treatment of noncognitive behavioral disturbances in elderly demented patients. *American Journal of Psychiatry* **147**, 1640–1645.

Stein, G. (1994) Physical treatments of the personality disorders. *Current Opinion in Psychiatry* **7**, 129–136.

Yudofsky, S.C., Silver, J.M. and Hales, R.E. (1990) Pharmacologic management of aggression in the elderly. *Journal of Clinical Psychiatry* **51**, (suppl.10), 22–28.

Eating Disorders

Fettes, P.A. and Peters, J.M. (1992) A meta-analysis of group treatments for bulimia nervosa. *International Journal of Eating Disorders* **11**, 97–110.

Garfinkel, P.E. and Goldbloom, D.S. (1993) Bulimia nervosa: a review of therapy research. *Journal of Psychotherapy and Practical Research* **2**, 38–50.

Garrow, J.S. (1992) Treatment of obesity. *Lancet* **340**, 409–413.

Goldstein, D.J. (1992) Beneficial health effects of modest weight loss. *International Journal of Obesity* **16**, 397–415.

Hartmann, A., Herzog, T. and Drinkmann, A. (1992) Psychotherapy of bulimia nervosa: what is effective? A meta-analysis. *Journal of Psychosomatic Research* **36**, 159–167.

Kennedy, S.H. and Goldbloom, D.S. (1994) Advances in the treatment of anorexia nervosa and bulimia nervosa. *CNS Drugs* **1**, 201–212.

Laessle, R.G., Zoettl, C. and Pirke, P.M. (1987) Meta-analysis of treatment studies for bulimia. *International Journal of Eating Disorders* **6**, 647–653.

Oesterheld, J.R., McKenna, M.S. and Gould, N.B. (1987) Group psychotherapy of bulimia: a critical review. *International Journal of Group Psychotherapy* **37**, 163.

Saris, W.H.M. (1993) The role of exercise in the dietary treatment of obesity. *International Journal of Obesity* **17**, S17–S21.

Silverstone, T. (1992) Appetite suppressants. A review. *Drugs*, **43**, 820–836.

Weintraub, M. (ed.) (1992) Long-term weight control: the National Heart, Lung, and Blood Institute funded multimodal intervention study. *Clinical Pharmacology and Therapeutics* **51** (suppl.), 581–646.

Epilepsy

Bauer, J. and Alger, C.E. (1994) Management of status epilepticus in adults. *CNS Drugs* **1**, 26–44.

Dodrill, C.B. (1992) Problems in the assessment of cognitive effects of antiepileptic drugs. *Epilepsia* **33** (suppl. 6), 29–32.

Fenwick, P.B.C. (1992) The relationship between mind, brain, and seizures. *Epilepsia* **33** (suppl. 6), 1–6.

Goa, K.L., Ross, S.R. and Chrisp, P. (1993) Lamotrigine. A review of its pharmacological properties and clinical efficacy in epilepsy. *Drugs* **46**, 152–176.

Meador, K.J., Loring, D.W., Huh, K., Gallagher, B.B. and King, D.W. (1990) Comparative cognitive effects of anticonvulsants. *Neurology* **40**, 391–394.

Nichols, M.E., Meader, K.J. and Loring, D.W. (1993) Neuropsychological effects of antiepileptic drugs: a current perspective. *Clinical Neuropharmacology* **16**, 471–484.
Thompson, P.J. (1992) Antiepileptic drugs and memory. *Epilepsia* **33** (suppl. 6), 37–40.

Reproduction

Schou, M. (1990) Lithium treatment during pregnancy, delivery, and lactation: an update. *Journal of Clinical Psychiatry* **51**, 410–413.
Young, R.L. and Goldzieher, J.W. (1987) Current status of postmenopausal oestrogen therapy. *Drugs* **33**, 95–106.

INDEX

The Wiley Series in

CLINICAL PSYCHOLOGY

Related titles of interest from Wiley...

Multiple Selves, Multiple Voices
Working with Trauma, Violation and Dissociation
Phil Mollon

Shows how new understanding of trauma and dissociation can transform our view of many severe personality disturbances, including the extreme condition of Multiple Personality/Dissociative Identity Disorder (MPD/DID).

0471 95292 3   232pp   1996   Hardback
0471 96330 5   232pp   1996   Paperback

Obsessive Compulsive Disorder
A Cognitive and Neuropsychological Perspective
Frank Tallis

Reviews the nature and incidence of OCD in light of the related research on cognitive processes and cognitive neuropsychology, with special reference to treatment using behavioural and cognitive therapies.

0471 95775 5   222pp   1995   Hardback
0471 95772 0   222pp   1995   Paperback

Cognitive Behaviour Therapy for Psychosis
Theory and Practice
David Fowler, Philippa Garety and Elizabeth Kuipers

Focuses on the four main problems presented by people with psychosis: emotional disturbance; psychotic symptoms like delusions and bizarre beliefs; social disabilities; and relapse risk.

0471 93980 3   212pp   1995   Hardback
0471 95618 X   212pp   1995   Paperback

Psychological Management of Schizophrenia
Edited by Max Birchwood and Nicholas Tarrier

Offers a practical guide for mental health professionals wanting to develop and enhance their skills in new treatment approaches.

0471 95056 4   176pp   1994   Paperback